The Anti-Inflammatory Diet Cookbook for Lunch

Lots of Tasty Ideas for Your Lunches While Following the Anti-Inflammatory Diet

By
Olga Jones

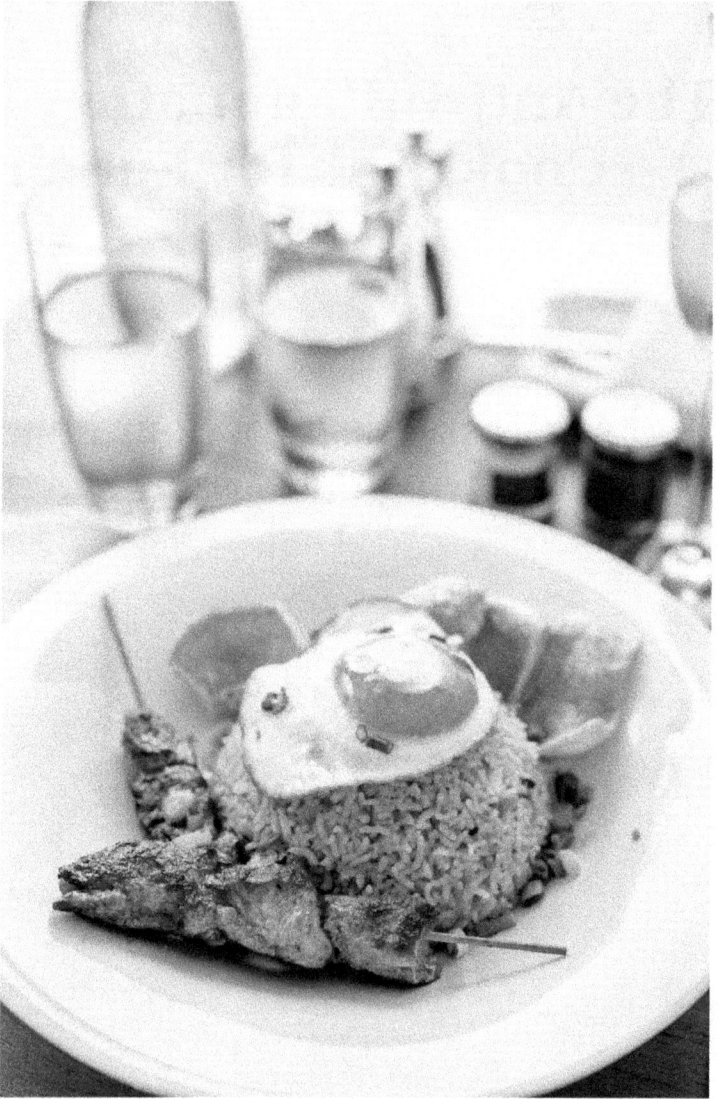

the publisher or the original author of this work can be in any fashion deemed liable for any hardship or damages that may befall them after undertaking information described herein.

Additionally, the information in the following pages is intended only for informational purposes and should thus be thought of as universal. As befitting its nature, it is presented without assurance regarding its prolonged validity or interim quality. Trademarks that are mentioned are done without written consent and can in no way be considered an endorsement from the trademark holder.

Table of Contents

INTRODUCTION

What is the Anti-Inflammatory Diet?

The anti-inflammatory diet is the best choice for your health if you have conditions that cause inflammation. Such conditions are asthma, chronic peptic ulcer, tuberculosis, rheumatoid arthritis, periodontitis, Crohn's disease, sinusitis, active hepatitis, etc. Along with medical treatment, proper nutrition is very important. An anti-inflammatory diet can help to reduce the pain from inflammation for a few notches. Such a diet isn't a panacea but a significant help in any treatment. Inflammation is a natural response of your body to infections, injuries, and illnesses. The classic symptoms of inflammation are redness, pain, heat, and swelling. Nevertheless, some diseases don't have any symptoms. Such illnesses are diabetes, heart disease, cancer, etc. That's why we should care about our health permanently and an anti-inflammatory diet is one of the ways for it.

Inflammation is your immune system's response to injury or unwanted microbes in your body. It is a natural process and vital part of your body's healing process. When inflammation becomes systemic and chronic, however, it becomes a problem, and measures need to be taken. This type of inflammation serves no purpose, and can cause a lot of harm to the body.

This book has a LOT of recipes, and not every recipe might work for you. For example, if you're allergic to dairy or gluten, the recipes containing those ingredients will cause more harm than good. However, substitutions are possible for all of these, so you will be fine following this book as long as you keep an eye on the ingredients and use a bit of creativity where you have to! Once you understand the fundamentals of the diet, you will be fully equipped to create your own recipes from scratch!This is the most important information that you should know before starting a diet. Any diet is not a magic remedy for all diseases; it is a support for the body during a difficult time of treatment. Start your new healthy life from one small step and you will see the huge results within half a year. You can be sure that your body will be thankful to you by giving you a fresh look and energy for new achievements.

Curried Carrot & Sweet Potato Soup

Yield: 5 servings
Preparation Time: fifteen minutes
Cooking Time: 37 minutes

Ingredients:
- 2 teaspoons olive oil
- ½ cup shallots, chopped
- 1½ cups carrots, peeled and sliced into ¼-inch size
- 3 cups sweet potato, peeled and cubed into ½-inch size
- 1 tablespoon fresh ginger, grated
- 2 teaspoons curry powder
- 3 cups Fat-free chicken broth
- Salt, to taste

Directions:
1. In a sizable soup pan, heat oil on medium heat.
2. Add shallots and sauté for approximately 3 minutes.
3. Add carrot, sweet potato, ginger and curry powder and sauté for around 3-4 minutes.
4. Add broth and bring to a boil.Reduce heat to low.
5. Cover and simmer approximately 25-thirty minutes.
6. Stir in salt and black pepper and remove from heat.
7. Keep aside to cool down the slightly.
8. In a blender, add soup in batches and pulse till smooth.
9. Serve immediately.

Pumpkin Soup

Yield: 2 servings
Preparation Time: quarter-hour
Cooking Time: 18 minutes

Ingredients:
- 2 teaspoons coconut oil
- 1 brown onion, chopped
- 1 (¾-inch) fresh turmeric piece
- 1 (¾-inch) fresh galangal piece
- 1 long red chili, seeded and chopped
- 2 tablespoons fresh cilantro, chopped
- 4 kefir lime leaves
- 3 cups pumpkin, peeled and cubed
- 1 teaspoon fresh lime peel piece
- 1 large garlic oil, chopped
- 4 cups vegetable broth
- 2 tablespoons fish sauce
- ½ cup coconut cream
- 2 tablespoons fresh lime juice

Directions:
1. In a substantial soup pan, heat oil on medium heat.
2. Add onion, turmeric, galangal, red chili, cilantro and lime leaves and sauté for approximately 2-3 minutes.
3. Add pumpkin, lime peel, garlic, broth and fish sauce and convey to your boil. Reduce the heat to low.
4. Cover and simmer approximately quarter hour.
5. Remove from heat whilst aside to chill slightly.
6. Discard the turmeric, galangal and lemon peel.

7. In a blender, add soup mixture with coconut cream and lemon juice in batches and pulse till smooth.

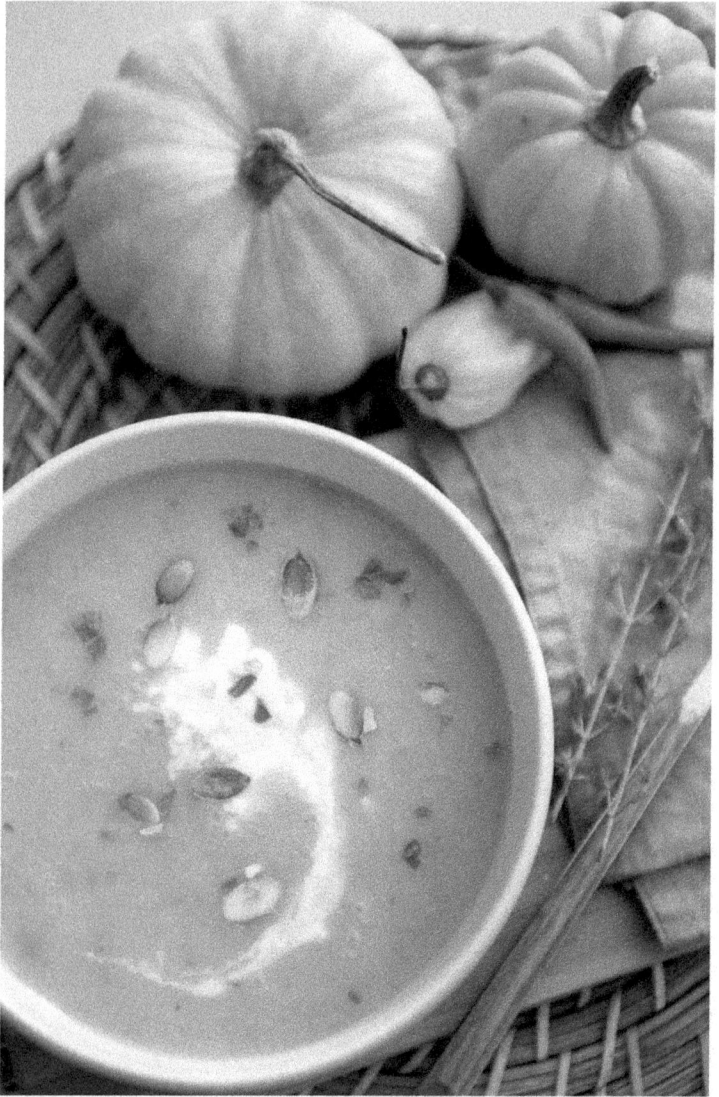

Butternut Squash Soup

Yield: 4 servings
Preparation Time: quarter-hour
Cooking Time: twenty minutes

Ingredients:
- 1 small butternut squash, peeled, seeded and cubed
- 2 tablespoons coconut oil, melted
- Salt, to taste
- 4 cups reduced-sodium vegetable broth, divided
- 14- ounces coconut milk
- 1 small shallot, sliced thinly
- 2 lemongrass stalks, cut into 6-inch pieces
- 3 tablespoons fresh ginger, grated
- ½ of Serrano pepper, chopped
- 1 cup fresh mushrooms, sliced
- Freshly ground black pepper, to taste
- 2 tablespoons fresh lime juice
- Chopped fresh cilantro, for garnishing

Directions:
1. Preheat the oven to 400 degrees F.
2. Place the butternut squash in a baking sheet.
3. Drizzle with oil and sprinkle with salt and roast approximately 12- quarter-hour.
4. Remove from oven whilst aside to chill completely.
5. In a big soup pan, add 3 cups from the broth, coconut milk, shallot, lemongrass, ginger and Serrano pepper and bring to a boil. Reduce the warmth to simmer.
6. In a blender, add roasted butternut squash and remaining broth and pulse till smooth.

7. Add squash puree and mushrooms in simmering broth and stir to combine.

8. Simmer for about 5 minutes.

9. Stir in salt, black pepper and lime juice and take away from heat.

10. Serve hot with all the garnishing of cilantro.

Cauliflower & Zucchini Soup

Yield: 4-6 servings
Preparation Time: quarter-hour
Cooking Time: 45 minutes

Ingredients:

- 2-3 cups cauliflower, chopped into large pieces
- 2 tablespoons coconut oil, divided
- 1 medium yellow onion, chopped
- 1 tablespoon garlic, minced
- 1 teaspoon fresh ginger, minced
- 1 teaspoon dried ginger
- 1½ teaspoons ground coriander
- Salt and freshly ground black pepper, to taste
- 1½ pound zucchini, peeled and chopped
- 4 cups chicken broth
- ½ cup coconut milk
- Chopped chives, for garnishing

Directions:

1. Preheat the oven to 375 degrees F.
2 Place the cauliflower in a baking sheet and drizzle with 1 tablespoon of oil
3. Roast approximately half an hour, stirring once in the middle way.
4. Meanwhile in a large soup pan, heat remaining oil on medium heat.
5. Add onion and sauté approximately 5 minutes.
6. Add garlic, ginger, coriander, salt and black pepper and sauté for around 1 minute.
7. Add zucchini and cook for around 1 minute.

8. Add broth and produce to your boil.Reduce the temperature to simmer.

9. Add the cauliflower and stir to combine.

10. Simmer approximately quarter-hour.

11. Remove in the heat and stir in coconut milk.

12. With an immersion blender, puree the soup completely.

13. Serve hot with the topping of chives.

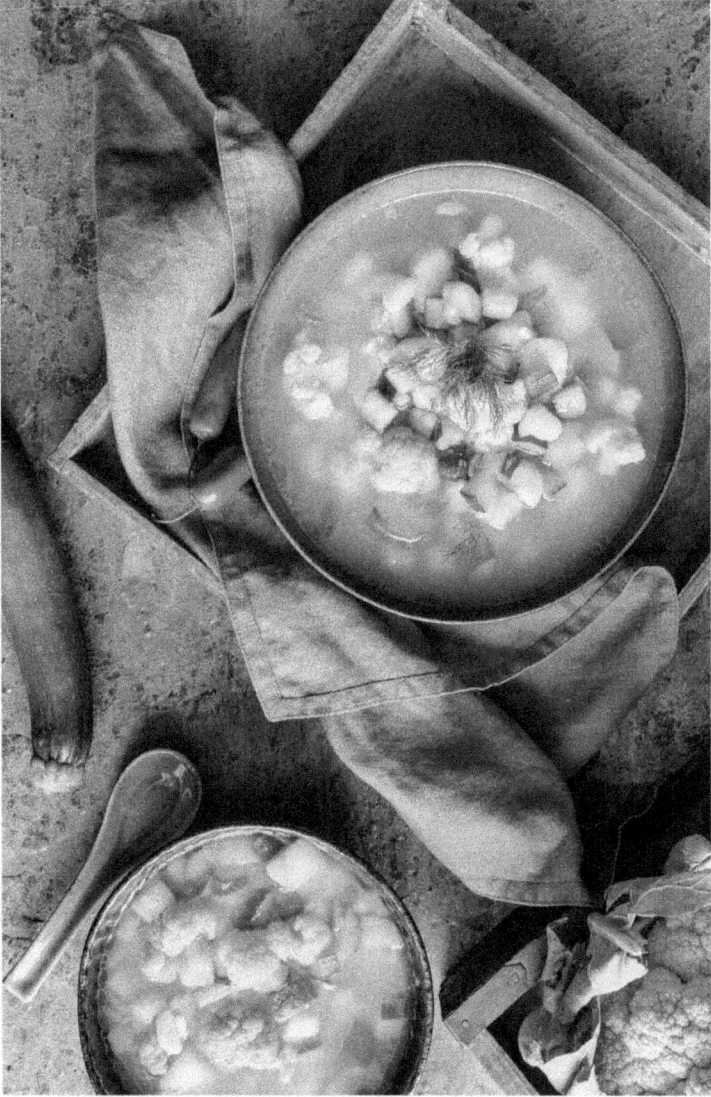

Kabocha Squash Soup

Yield: 8 servings
Preparation Time: quarter-hour
Cooking Time: 65 minutes

Ingredients:
- 1 (4-5-pound) kabocha squash, stemmed, peeled, seeded and chopped
- Coconut oil, as required
- 1 large sweet onion, chopped
- 6-10 garlic cloves, chopped
- 6 cups chicken broth
- 1 (14-ounce) can coconut milk
- ¼ teaspoon ground cumin
- ¼ teaspoon ground ginger
- ¼ teaspoon ground turmeric
- Pinch of freshly ground white pepper
- Salt and freshly ground black pepper, to taste
- Pumpkin seeds, for garnishing

Directions:
1. Preheat the oven to 350 degrees F.
2. Place the squash into a baking sheet and drizzle with a few melted oil
3. Roast for around 30-45 minutes or till 10der.
4. Remove from oven and set aside.
5. In a substantial soup pan, heat some oil on medium heat.
6. Add onion and garlic and sauté for around 4-5 minutes.
7. Add squash and remaining ingredients and simmer approximately 10-15 minutes.

8. Remove from heat and by having an immersion blender, puree the soup completely.

9. Serve hot using the topping of pumpkin seeds.

Mixed Veggie Soup

Yield: 4 servings
Preparation Time: twenty or so minutes
Cooking Time: 31 minutes

Ingredients:
- 1 tbsp extra virgin olive oil
- ½ of small onion, chopped
- 1 tablespoon fresh ginger herb, chopped finely
- 2-3 garlic cloves, minced
- ¼ teaspoon ground turmeric
- 2 celery stalks, chopped
- ½ head of cauliflower, chopped
- 2 small potatoes, peeled and chopped
- 2 large carrots, peeled and chopped
- 1 medium zucchini, chopped
- Salt and freshly ground black pepper, to taste
- 2 tablespoons fresh lemon juice
- ¼-½ teaspoon cayenne
- 4 cups vegetable broth

Directions:
1. In a substantial soup pan, heat oil on medium heat.
2. Add onion, ginger, garlic and turmeric and sauté for approximately 4-5 minutes.
3. Add vegetables, salt and black pepper and cook, stirring occasionally approximately 5-7 minutes.
4. Stir in fresh lemon juice.
5. Add red pepper cayenne and broth and produce to a boil.
6. Simmer, covered for about 10-15 minutes.

7. Remove from heat and with an immersion blender, puree the soup completely.

8. Return the soup in pan on medium-low heat and simmer for around 3-4 minutes or till heated completely.

9. Serve immediately.

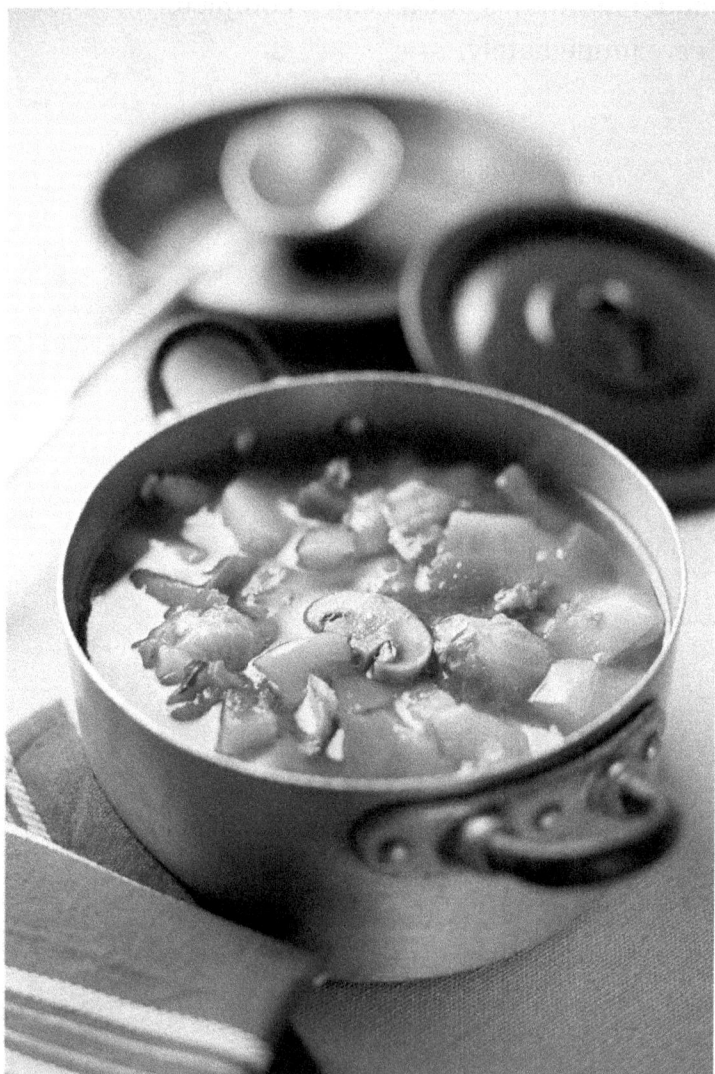

Roasted Sweet Potato

Yield: 2-3 servings
Preparation Time: 15 minutes
Cooking Time: twenty minutes

Ingredients:
- 1 teaspoon coconut oil
- 1 onion, chopped
- 2 medium sweet potatoes, peeled and cubed
- ½ tablespoon ground turmeric
- 1-2 fresh parsley sprigs
- Salt and freshly ground black pepper, to taste
- Water, as required

Directions:
1. In a skillet, melt coconut oil on low heat.
2. Add onion and sauté approximately 810 minutes.
3. Stir in sweet potato turmeric, parsley, salt and black pepper.
4. Add enough water that covers the sweet potato midway.
5. Cook for around 68 minutes or till desired doneness.

Roasted Summer Squash & Fennel Bulb

Yield: 4 servings
Preparation Time: quarter-hour
Cooking Time: fifteen minutes

Ingredients:

- 2 small summer squash, cubed into 1-inch size
- 1½ cups fennel bulb, sliced
- 1 tablespoon fresh thyme, chopped
- 1 tablespoon extra-virgin organic olive oil
- Salt and freshly ground black pepper, to taste
- ¼ cup garlic, sliced thinly
- 1 tablespoon fennel fronds, chopped

Directions:

1. Preheat the oven to 450 degrees F.
2. In a substantial bowl, add all ingredients except garlic and fennel fronds and toss to coat well.
3. Transfer a combination right into a large rimmed baking sheet.
4. Roast for approximately 10 min.
5. Remove from oven and stir in sliced garlic.
6. Roast for 5 minutes more.
7. Remove from oven and stir inside the fennel fronds.
8. Serve immediately

Potato Mash

Yield: 32 servings
Preparation Time: fifteen minutes
Cooking Time: 20 minutes

Ingredients:
- 10 large baking potatoes, peeled and cubed
- 3 tablespoons organic olive oil, divided
- 1 onion, chopped
- 1 tablespoon ground turmeric
- ½ teaspoon ground cumin
- Salt and freshly ground black pepper, to taste

Directions:
1. In a large pan of water, add potatoes and produce with a boil on medium-high heat.
2. Cook for approximately twenty or so minutes.
3. Drain well and transfer into a large bowl.
4. With a potato masher, mash the potatoes.
5. Meanwhile in a very skillet, heat 1 tablespoon of oil on medium-high heat.
6. Add onion and sauté for about 6 minutes.
7. Add onion mixture in the bowl with mashed potatoes.
8. Add turmeric, cumin, salt and black pepper and mash till well combined.
9. Stir in remaining oil and serve.

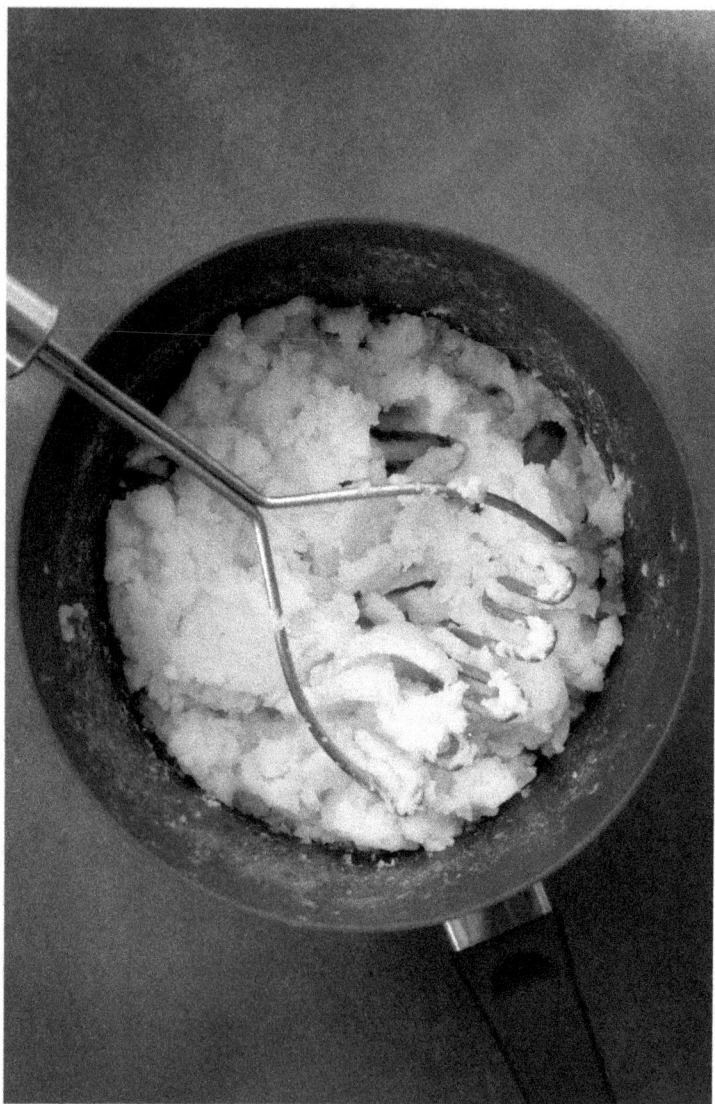

Gingered Cauliflower Rice

Yield: 3-4 servings
Preparation Time: quarter-hour
Cooking Time: 10 minutes

Ingredients:
- 3 tablespoons coconut oil
- 4 (1/8-inch thick) fresh ginger slices
- 1 small head cauliflower, trimmed and processed into rice consis10cy
- 3 garlic cloves, crushed
- 1 tablespoon chives, chopped
- 1 tablespoon coconut vinegar
- Salt, to taste

Directions:
1. In a skillet, melt coconut oil on medium-high heat.
2. Add ginger and sauté for about 2-3 minutes.
3. Discard the ginger slices and stir in cauliflower and garlic.
4. Cook, stirring occasionally approximately 7-8 minutes.
5. Stir in remaining ingredients and take off from heat.
6. Serve immediately

Simple Brown Rice

Yield: 4 servings
Preparation Time: 10 min
Cooking Time: 50 minutes

Ingredients:

- 1 cup brown rice
- 2 cups chicken broth
- 1 tablespoon ground turmeric
- 1 tbsp extra virgin olive oil

Directions:

1. In a pan, add rice, broth and turmeric and provide with a boil.
2. Reduce the warmth to low.
3. Simmer, covered for about 50 minutes.
4. Add the organic olive oil and fluff using a fork.
5. Keep aside, covered approximately 10 minutes before serving.

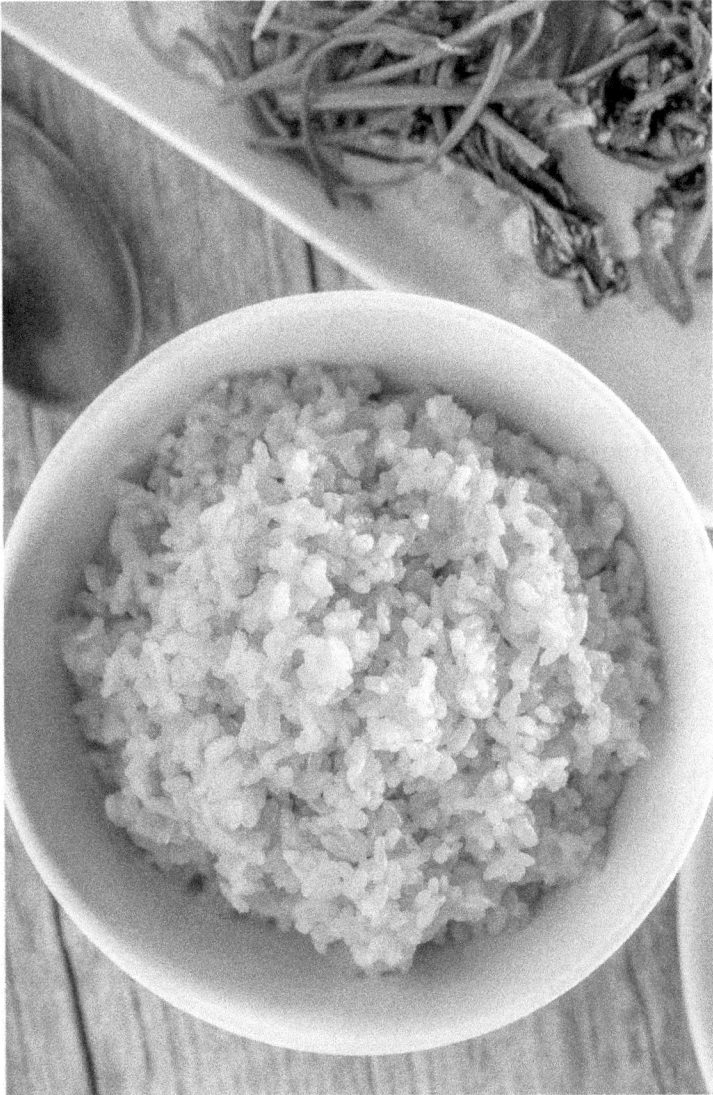

Quinoa With Apricots

Yield: 4 servings
Preparation Time: 15 minutes
Cooking Time: 12 minutes

Ingredients:

- 2 cups water
- 1 cup quinoa
- ½ teaspoon fresh ginger, grated finely
- ½ cup dried apricots, chopped roughly
- Salt and freshly ground black pepper, to taste

Directions:

1. In a pan, add water on high heat and bring to your boil.

2. Add quinoa and reduce the heat to medium.

3. Cover and reduce the heat to low.

4. Simmer for about 12 minutes.

5. Remove from heat and immediately, stir in ginger and apricots.

6. Keep aside, covered for approximately fifteen minutes before serving.

Grilled Veggie Skewers

Yield: 5 servings
Preparation Time: 20 minutes
Cooking Time: fifteen minutes

Ingredients:
For Marinade Mixture:

- 3 garlic cloves, chopped
- 1 (1-inch) pieces fresh ginger, chopped
- 1 teaspoon ground cumin
- 1 teaspoon ground coriander
- 1teaspoon sweet paprika
- 1/8 teaspoon red chili powder
- Salt and freshly ground black pepper, to taste
- ¼ cup fresh lemon juice
- ¼ cup organic olive oil
- ½ lot of fresh cilantro
- ½ couple of fresh parsley

For Vegetables:

- 2 medium red bell pepper, seeded and cut into 1-inch pieces
- 2 medium zucchinis, cut into 1/3-inch thick round slices
- 1 pound small mushrooms
- 1 large yellow onion, sliced into 1-inch pieces
- 1 large eggplant, quartered lengthwise and cut into ½-inch thick slices diagonally

Directions:
1. For marinade mixture in the blender, add all ingredients except herbs and pulse till well combined.

2. Add fresh herbs and pulse till smooth.

3. In a sizable bowl, add vegetables and marinade and toss to coat well.

4. Refrigerate, covered approximately 4 hours.

5. Preheat the grill to medium-low heat. Grease the grill grate.

6. Thread the skewers for around 15 minutes, flipping occasionally.

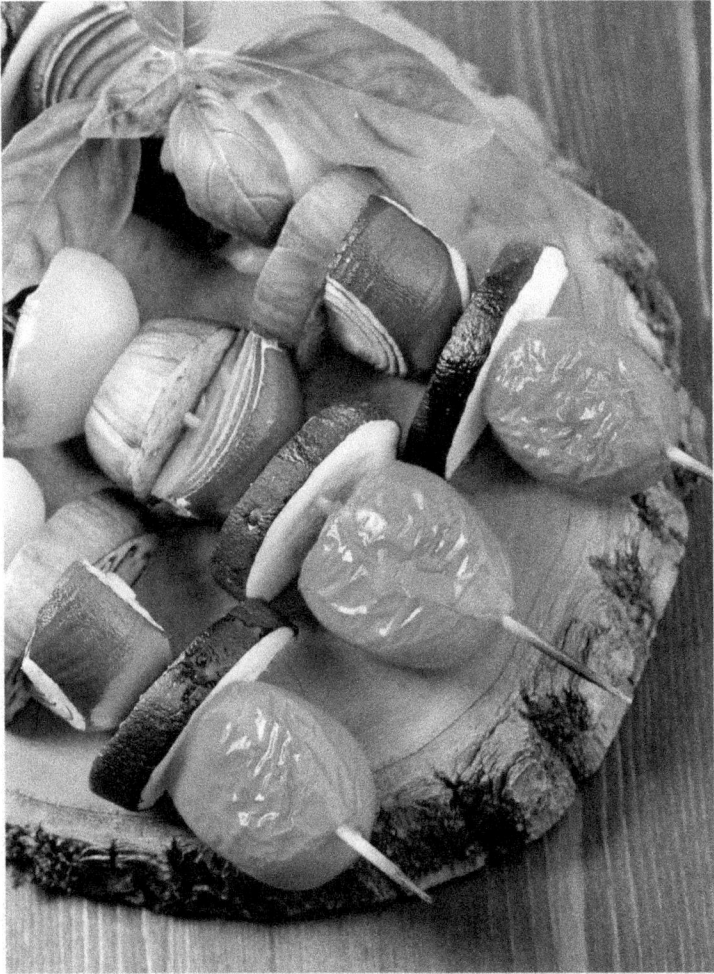

Three Mushrooms Medley

Yield: 3 servings
Preparation Time: 15 minutes
Cooking Time: 17 minutes

Ingredients:
- 3 tablespoons extra-virgin extra virgin olive oil
- 3 portabella mushrooms, sliced
- 6-ounce shiitake mushrooms, stemmed and sliced
- 7½-ounce baby beech mushrooms
- 1 tablespoon fresh ginger, minced
- 5 garlic cloves, minced
- 1 dried red chili, crushed
- 2 teaspoons coconut aminos
- 1 teaspoon sesame oil

Directions:
1. In a skillet, heat 1 tablespoon of essential olive oil on medium heat.
2. Add portabella mushrooms and cook stirring occasionally for approximately 4-5 minutes. Transfer the mushrooms in a large bowl.
3. In a similar skillet, heat 1 tablespoon of extra virgin olive oil on medium heat.
4. Add shiitake mushrooms and cook for approximately 4-5 minutes.
5. Transfer the mushrooms into the large bowl with portabella mushrooms.
6. In a similar skillet, heat ½ tablespoon from the organic olive oil on medium heat.

7. Add baby beech mushrooms and cook approximately 3-4 minutes.

8. Transfer the mushrooms to the large bowl with portabella mushrooms.

9. In exactly the same skillet, heat remaining extra virgin olive oil on medium heat.

10. Add ginger, garlic and red chili and sauté for around 1 minute.

11. Add the mushroom mixture, coconut aminos and sesame oil and stir till well combined.

12. Cook for around 1-2 minutes.

13. Serve hot.

Nutty Spinach

Yield: 4 servings
Preparation Time: fifteen minutes
Cooking Time: 23 minutes

Ingredients:
- 3 tablespoons coconut oil
- 1½ tablespoons coconut sugar
- ½ teaspoon cumin seeds
- 1 tablespoon black mustard seeds
- ¼ teaspoon fenugreek seeds
- 2 pounds fresh spinach, trimmed
- 1 tablespoon green chili, minced
- ½ tablespoon fresh ginger, grated
- 2/3 cup almonds, soaked in warm water for 4 hours and drained
- 1/3 cup coconut, shredded
- Salt and freshly ground black pepper, to taste
- 2 tablespoons water
- 1/8 teaspoon ground nutmeg

Directions:
1. In a big skillet, melt coconut oil on medium heat.
2. Add brown sugar, cumin seeds, mustard seeds and fenugreek seeds and sauté for around 1 minute.
3. Stir in spinach, green chili, ginger, almonds, coconut, salt and black pepper.
4. Reduce the heat to low and simmer, covered approximately 10 minutes.
5. Uncover and stir in water and simmer approximately 10 min.

6. Stir within the nutmeg and simmer for about 1-2 minutes more.

Mixed Vegetables Stew

Yield: 4 servings
Preparation Time: 20 min
Cooking Time: 52 minutes

Ingredients:
- 2 tablespoons organic olive oil
- 1¼ cups yellow onion, chopped
- 1 tablespoon garlic, minced
- 1 tablespoon chile paste
- 1½ tablespoons fresh turmeric, grated
- 1½ teaspoons ground cumin
- 1 teaspoon ground cinnamon
- 1 cup carrots, peeled and chopped roughly
- 1 cup cauliflower, chopped roughly
- 2 cups broccoli, chopped roughly
- 4 cups green cabbage, chopped roughly
- 1 cup coconut water
- 2 cups canned crushed tomatoes
- ¾ cup frozen peas, thawed
- Salt and freshly ground black pepper, to taste

Directions:
1. In a sizable pan, heat oil on medium heat.
2. Add onion and garlic and sauté approximately 10 min.
3. Add chile paste, turmeric, cumin and cinnamon and saute for around 1 minute.
4. Stir in carrots and cook for around 3-4 minutes.
5. Stir in cauliflower and broccoli and cook for about 2-3 minutes.
6. Stir in cabbage reducing heat to low.

7. Simmer for about 4 minutes.

8. Add coconut water and tomatoes and produce to some boil on medium-high heat.

9. Reduce heat to low and simmer, covered for approximately thirty minutes.

10. Stir in peas, salt and black pepper and remove from heat.

11. Serve hot.

Veggies Curry in Pumpkin Puree

Yield: 4 servings
Preparation Time: fifteen minutes
Cooking Time: a half-hour

Ingredients:
- 1 tablespoon coconut oil
- 1 green bell pepper, seeded and chopped
- 1 onion, chopped
- 1 cup homemade pumpkin puree
- 1 tablespoon curry powder
- 1 teaspoon ground cinnamon
- ¼ teaspoon ground ginger
- Salt, to taste
- 1 (14- ounce) can coconut milk
- 1 cup water
- 1 sweet potato, peeled and cut into 1- inch cubes
- 1 head broccoli, cut into florets

Directions:
1. In a big pan, melt coconut oil on medium heat.
2. Add onion and sauté for about 8 minutes.
3. Add pumpkin puree, curry powder, cinnamon, ginger, salt, coconut milk and water and stir to blend well.
4. Stir in pumpkin and broccoli and bring with a gentle simmer.
5. Simmer, covered approximately 15-twenty minutes.
6. Serve hot.

Stuffed Zucchini

Yield: 6 servings
Preparation Time: twenty minutes
Cooking Time: half an hour

Ingredients

- 6 medium zucchinis, halved lengthwise
- Salt, to taste
- 1½ baking potatoes, peeled and cubed
- 4 teaspoons olive oil
- 2½ cups onion, chopped
- 1 Serrano chile, mined
- 2 minced garlic cloves
- 1½ tablespoons fresh ginger, minced
- 2 tablespoons chickpea flour
- 1 teaspoon ground coriander
- ¼ teaspoon ground cumin
- ¼ teaspoon ground turmeric
- Freshly ground black pepper, to taste
- 1½ cups frozen green peas, thawed
- 2 tablespoons fresh cilantro, chopped

Directions:

1. Preheat the oven to 375 degrees F.
2. With a scooper, scoop your pulp from zucchini halves, leaving about a ¼-inch thick shell.
3. In a shallow roasting pan, arrange the zucchini halves, cut side up.
4. Sprinkle the zucchini halves with a little salt.
5. In a pan of boiling water, cook the potatoes for around 2 minutes.

6. Drain well whilst aside.

7. In a nonstick skillet, heat oil on medium high heat.

8. Add onion, Serrano, garlic and dinger and sauté for around 3 minutes.

9. Reduce the heat to medium-low.

10. Stir in chickpea flour and spices and cook for about 5 minutes.

11. Stir in cooked potato, green peas and cilantro and take off from heat.

12. With a paper towel, pat dry the zucchini halves.

13. Stuff the zucchini halves with all the veggie mixture evenly.

14. Bake, covered for about twenty or so minutes.

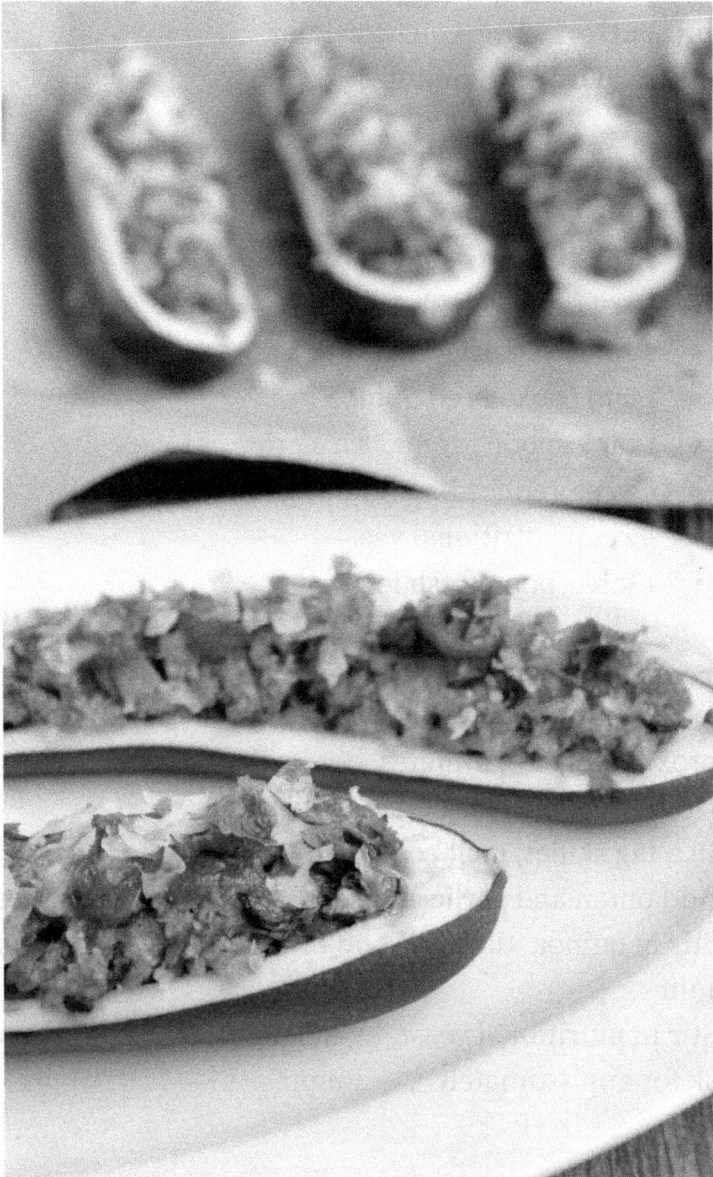

Quinoa with Asparagus

Yield: 4 servings
Preparation Time: quarter-hour
Cooking Time: 18 minutes

Ingredients:
- 1 pound fresh asparagus, trimmed
- 2 teaspoons coconut oil
- ½ of onion, chopped
- 2 minced garlic cloves
- 1 cup cooked red quinoa
- 1 tablespoon ground turmeric
- ½ cup reduced-sodium vegetable broth
- ½ cup nutritional yeast
- 1 tablespoon fresh lemon juice

Directions:
1. In a large pan of boiling water, cook the asparagus approximately 2-3 minutes.
2. Drain well and rinse under cold water.
3. In a big skillet, melt coconut oil on medium heat.
4. Add onion and garlic and sauté for around 5 minutes.
5. Stir in quinoa, turmeric and broth and cook for around 5-6 minutes.
6. Stir in nutritional yeast, fresh lemon juice and asparagus and cook for approximately 3-4 minutes.

Coconut Brown Rice

Yield: 14 servings
Preparation Time: fifteen minutes
Cooking Time: an hour

Ingredients:

- 12 cups water
- 1 tablespoon dried turmeric
- 2 pound brown rice
- 2 (13½- ounce) cans lite coconut milk
- 2 (13½-ounce) cans coconut milk
- 1 tablespoon fresh ginger, minced
- 1½ teaspoons fresh lemon zest, grated finely
- 4 dried bay leaves
- Salt and freshly ground black pepper, to taste
- Chopped cashews, for garnishing
- Chopped fresh cilantro, for garnishing

Directions:

1. In a small bowl, add water and turmeric and beat till well combined.
2. In a big pan, add turmeric water and remaining ingredients except cashews and stir well.
3. Bring with a boil on high heat.
4. Reduce heat to medium and simmer, stirring occasionally for about 30-35 minutes.
5. Reduce the temperature to low and simmer, covered for about 20-25 minutes.
6. Remove bay leaf before serving.
7. Garnish with cashews and cilantro and serve.

Brown Rice Casserole

Yield: 2 servings
Preparation Time: quarter-hour
Cooking Time: 60 minutes

Ingredients:

- 1 teaspoon extra-virgin olive oil
- 1 red onion, sliced thinly
- 1½ teaspoons ground turmeric
- 9-ounce brown mushrooms, sliced
- 1 teaspoon raisins
- ½ cup brown rice, rinsed
- 1¼ cups vegetable broth
- ¼ cup fresh cilantro, chopped
- ½ tablespoons pine nuts, toasted
- 1 tablespoon fresh lemon juice
- Salt and freshly ground black pepper, to taste

Directions:

1. Preheat the oven to 400 degrees F.
2. In an ovenproof casserole, heat oil on medium heat.
3. Add onion and turmeric and sauté for about 3 minutes.
4. Add mushrooms and stir fry for approximately 2 minutes.
5. Stir in raisins, rice and broth and transfer into oven.
6. Bake for around 45-55 minutes or till desired doneness.
7. Just before serving, stir in remaining ingredients.

Herbed Bulgur Pilaf

Yield: 6 servings
Preparation Time: 20 minutes
Cooking Time: 35 minutes

Ingredients:
- 2 tablespoons extra-virgin organic olive oil
- 2 cups onion, chopped
- 1 garlic clove, minced
- 1½ cups medium bulgur
- ½ teaspoon ground cumin
- ½ teaspoon ground turmeric
- 1½ cups carrot, peeled and chopped
- 2 teaspoons fresh ginger, grated finely
- Salt, to taste
- 2 cups vegetable broth
- 3 tablespoons freshly squeezed lemon juice
- ¼ cup fresh parsley, chopped
- ¼ cup fresh mint leaves, chopped
- ¼ cup fresh dill, chopped
- ½ cup walnuts, toasted and chopped

Directions:
1. In a big deep skillet, heat oil on medium-low heat.
2. Add onion and cook, stirring occasionally for around 12-18 minutes.
3. Add garlic and sauté for about 1 minute.
4. Add bulgur, cumin and turmeric and stir fry for approximately 1 minute.
5. Add carrot, ginger, salt and broth and provide to a boil, stirring occasionally.

6. Simmer, covered for around quarter-hour.

7. Remove from heat and keep aside, covered for about 5 minutes.

8. Stir in fresh lemon juice and fresh herbs and serve while using garnishing of walnuts.

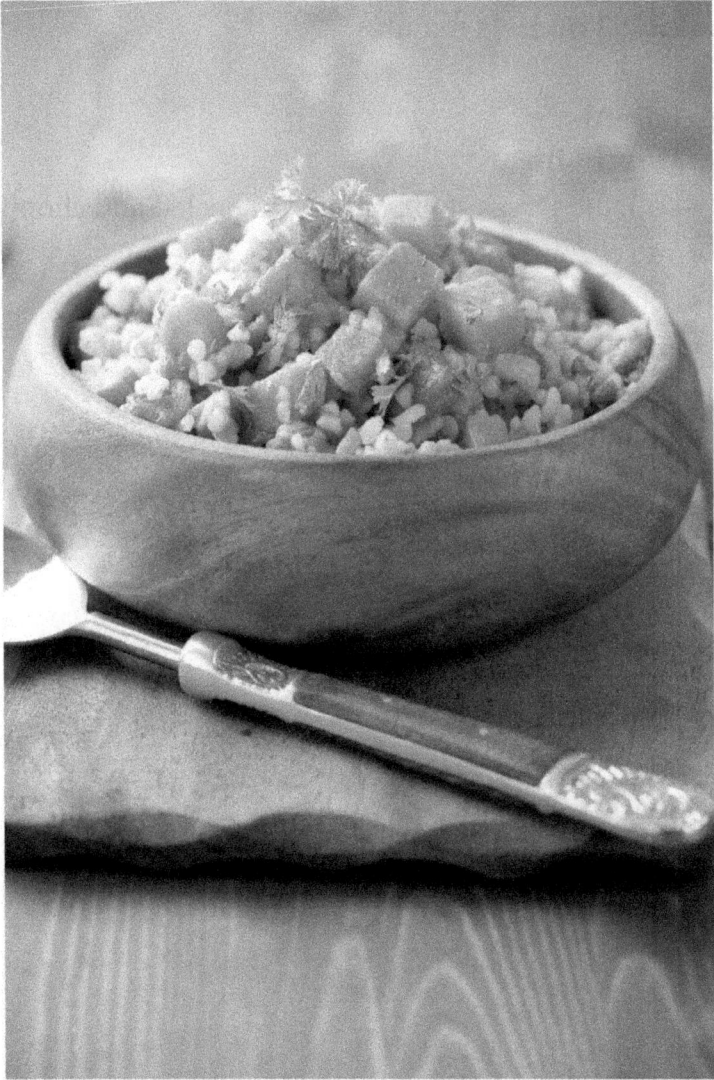

Baked Meatballs & Scallions

Yield: 4-6 servings
Preparation Time: 20 min
Cooking Time: 35 minutes

Ingredients:
For Meatballs:
- 1 lemongrass stalk, outer skin peeled and chopped
- 1 (1½-inch) piece fresh ginger, sliced
- 3 garlic cloves, chopped
- 1 cup fresh cilantro leaves, chopped roughly
- ½ cup fresh basil leaves, chopped roughly
- 2 tablespoons plus 1 teaspoon fish sauce
- 2 tablespoons water
- 2 tablespoons fresh lime juice
- ½ pound lean ground pork
- 1 pound lean ground lamb
- 1 carrot, peeled and grated
- 1 organic egg, bea10

For Scallions:
- 16 stalks scallions, trimmed
- 2 tablespoons coconut oil, melted
- Salt, to taste
- ½ cup water

Directions:
1. Preheat the oven to 375 degrees F. Grease a baking dish.
2. In a blender, add lemongrass, ginger, garlic, fresh herbs, fish sauce, water and lime juice and pulse till chopped finely.

3. Transfer the amalgamation in a bowl with remaining ingredients and mix till well combined.

4. Make about 1-inch balls from mixture.

5. Arrange the balls into prepared baking dish in a single layer.

6. In another rimmed baking dish, arrange scallion stalks in a very single layer.

7. Drizzle with coconut oil and sprinkle with salt.

8. Pour water in the baking dish 1nd with a foil paper cover it tightly.

9. Bake the scallion for around a half-hour.

10. Bake the meatballs for approximately 30-35 minutes. Pork with Bell Pepper This stir fry not simply tastes wonderful but additionally is packed with nutritious benefits.

Pork with Pineapple

Yield: 4 servings
Preparation Time: 15 minutes
Cooking Time: 14 minutes

Ingredients:
- 2 tablespoons coconut oil
- 1½ pound pork tenderloin, trimmed and cut into bite sized pieces
- 1 onion, chopped
- 2 minced garlic cloves
- 1 (1-inch) piece fresh ginger, minced
- 20-ounce pineapple, cut into chunks
- 1 large red bell pepper, seeded and chopped
- ¼ cup fresh pineapple juice
- ¼ cup coconut aminos
- Salt and freshly ground black pepper, to taste

Directions:
1. In a substantial skillet, melt coconut oil on high heat.
2. Add pork and stir fry approximately 4-5 minutes.
3. Transfer the pork right into a bowl.
4. In exactly the same skillet, heat remaining oil on medium heat.
5. Add onion, garlic and ginger and sauté for around 2 minutes.
6. Stir in pineapple and bell pepper and stir fry for around 3 minutes.
7. Stir in pork, pineapple juice and coconut aminos and cook for around 3-4 minutes.
8. Serve hot.

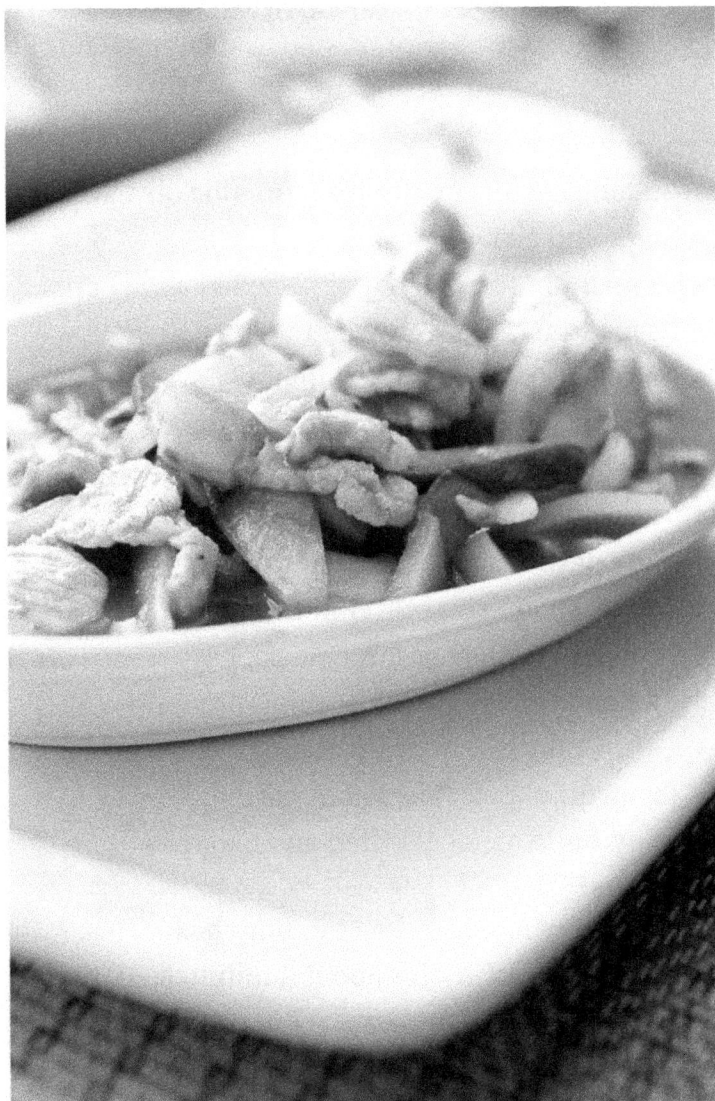

Pork Chili

Yield: 8 servings
Preparation Time: quarter-hour
Cooking Time: 60 minutes

Ingredients:
- 2 tablespoons extra-virgin organic olive oil
- 2 pound ground pork
- 1 medium red bell pepper, seeded and chopped
- 1 medium onion, chopped
- 5 garlic cloves, chopped finely
- 1 (2-inch) part of hot pepper, minced
- 1 tablespoon ground cumin
- 1 teaspoon ground turmeric
- 3 tablespoon chili powder
- ½ teaspoon chipotle chili powder
- Salt and freshly ground black pepper, to taste
- 1 cup chicken broth
- 1 (28-ounce) can fire-roasted crushed tomatoes
- 2 medium bok choy heads, sliced
- 1 avocado, peeled, pitted and chopped

Directions:
1. In a sizable pan, heat oil on medium heat.
2. Add pork and stir fry for about 5 minutes.
3. Add bell pepper, onion, garlic, hot pepper and spices and stir fry for approximately 5 minutes.
4. Add broth and tomatoes and convey with a boil.
5. Stir in bok choy and cook, covered for approximately twenty minutes.
6. Uncover and cook approximately 20-half an hour.
7. Serve hot while using topping of avocado.

Glazed Pork chops with Peach

Yield: 2 servings
Preparation Time: quarter-hour
Cooking Time: 16 minutes

Ingredients:

- 2 boneless pork chops
- Salt and freshly ground black pepper, to taste
- 1 ripe yellow peach, peeled, pitted, chopped and divided
- 1 tbsp organic olive oil
- 2 tablespoons shallot, minced
- 2 tablespoons garlic, minced
- 2 tablespoons fresh ginger, minced
- 1 tablespoon organic honey
- 1 tablespoon balsamic vinegar
- 1 tablespoon coconut aminos
- ¼ teaspoon red pepper flakes, crushed
- ¼ cup water

Directions:

1. Sprinkle the pork chops with salt and black pepper generously.
2. In a blender, add 1 / 2 of peach and pulse till a puree forms. Reserve remaining peach.
3. In a skillet, heat oil on medium heat.
4. Add shallots and sauté approximately 1-2 minutes.
5. Add garlic and ginger and sauté approximately 1 minute.
6. Add remaining ingredients and lower heat to medium-low.
7. Bring to your boil and simmer for approximately 4-5 minutes or till a sticky glaze forms.

8. Remove from heat and reserve 1/3 with the glaze and keep aside.

9. Coat the chops with remaining glaze.

10. Heat a nonstick skillet on medium-high heat.

11. Add chops and sear for around 4 minutes from both sides.

12. Transfer the chops in a plate and coat with all the remaining glaze evenly.

13. Top with reserved chopped peach and serve.

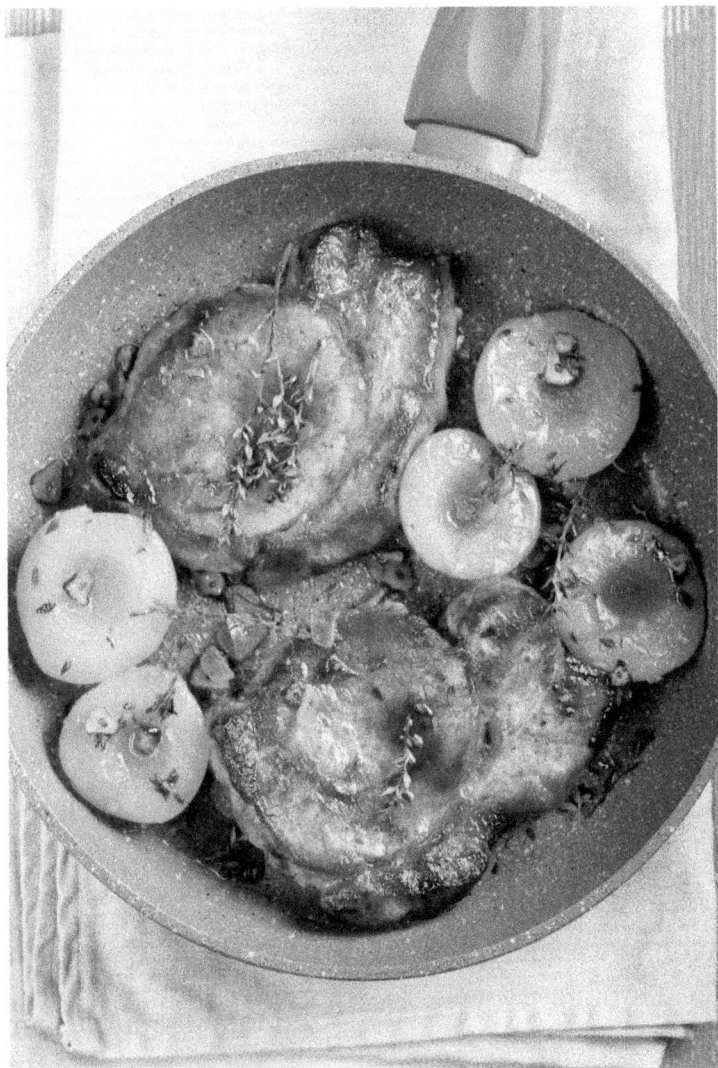

Baked Pork & Mushroom Meatballs

Yield: 6 servings
Preparation Time: 15 minutes
Cooking Time: fifteen minutes

Ingredients:
- 1 pound lean ground pork
- 1 organic egg white, bea10
- 4 fresh shiitake mushrooms, stemmed and minced
- 1 tablespoon fresh parsley, minced
- 1 tablespoon fresh basil leaves, minced
- 1 tablespoon fresh mint leaves, minced
- 2 teaspoons fresh lemon zest, grated finely
- 1½ teaspoons fresh ginger, grated finely
- Salt and freshly ground black pepper, to taste

Directions:
1. Preheat the oven to 425 degrees F. Arrange the rack inside the center of the oven.
2. Line a baking sheet with a parchment paper.
3. In a sizable bowl, add all ingredients and mix till well combined.
4. Make small equal-sized balls from mixture.
5. Arrange the balls onto prepared baking sheet in a single layer.
6. Bake for approximately 12-quarter-hour or till done completely.

Beef with Carrot & Broccoli

Yield: 4 servings
Preparation Time: fifteen minutes
Cooking Time: 14 minutes

Ingredients:
- 2 tablespoons coconut oil, divided
- 2 medium garlic cloves, minced
- 1 pound beef sirloin steak, trimmed and sliced into thin strips
- Salt, to taste
- ¼ cup chicken broth
- 2 teaspoons fresh ginger, grated
- 1 tablespoon ground flax seeds
- ½ teaspoon red pepper flakes, crushed
- ¼ teaspoon freshly ground black pepper
- 1 large carrot, peeled and sliced thinly
- 2 cups broccoli florets
- 1 medium scallion, sliced thinly

Directions:
1. In a substantial skillet, heat 1 tablespoon of oil on medium-high heat.
2. Add garlic and sauté approximately 1 minute.
3. Add beef and salt and cook for approximately 4-5 minutes or till browned.
4. With a slotted spoon, transfer the beef in a bowl.
5. Remove the liquid from skillet.
6. In a bowl, mix together broth, ginger, flax seeds, red pepper flakes and black pepper.
7. In a similar skillet, heat remaining oil on medium heat.

8. Add carrot, broccoli and ginger mixture and cook for approximately 3-4 minutes or till desired doneness.
9. Stir in beef and scallion and cook for around 3-4 minutes.

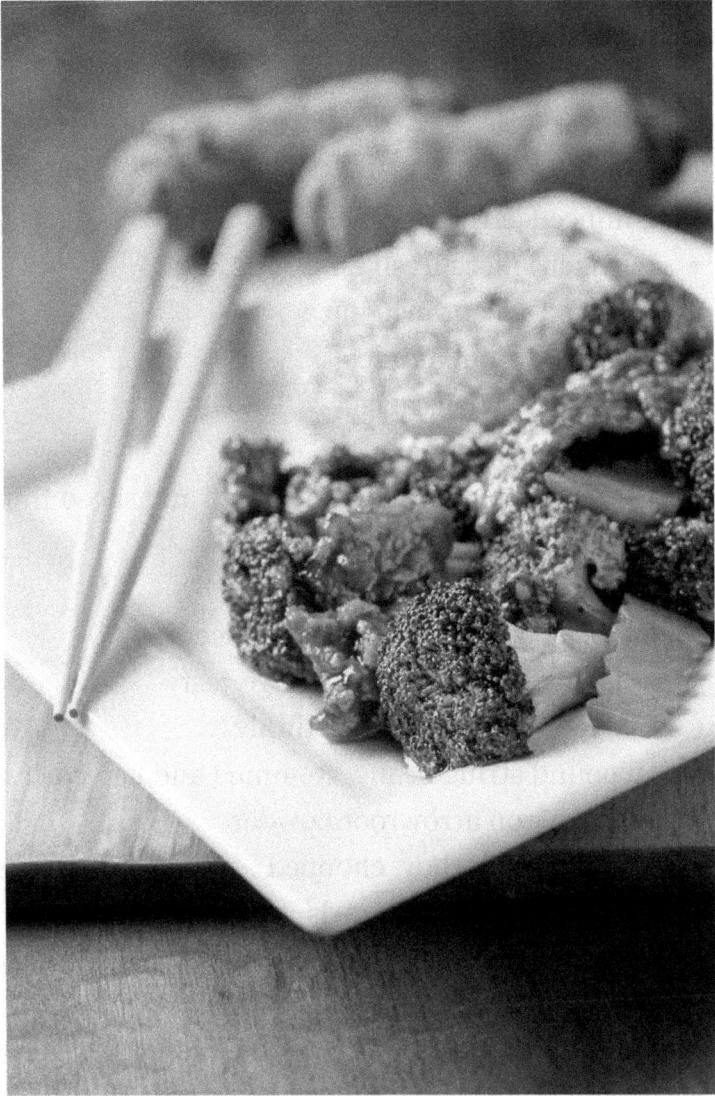

Citrus Beef with Bok Choy

Yield: 4 servings
Preparation Time: fifteen minutes
Cooking Time: 11 minutes

Ingredients:
For Marinade:
- 2 minced garlic cloves
- 1 (1-inch) piece fresh ginger, grated
- 1/3 cup fresh orange juice
- ½ cup coconut aminos
- 2 teaspoons fish sauce
- 2 teaspoons Sriracha
- 1¼ pound sirloin steak, trimmed and sliced thinly

For Veggies:
- 2 tablespoons coconut oil, divided
- 3-4 wide strips of fresh orange zest
- 1 jalapeño pepper, sliced thinly
- ½ pound string beans, stemmed and halved crosswise
- 1 tablespoon arrowroot powder
- ½ pound bok choy, chopped
- 2 teaspoons sesame seeds

Directions:
1. For marinade in a big bowl, mix together garlic, ginger, orange juice, coconut aminos, fish sauce and Sriracha.
2. Add beef and coat with marinade generously.
3. Refrigerate to marinate for around a couple of hours.
4. In a substantial skillet, heat oil on medium-high heat.
5. Add orange zest and sauté approximately 2 minutes.

6. Remove beef from bowl, reserving the marinade.

7. In the skillet, add beef and increase the heat to high.

8. Stir fry for about 2-3 minutes or till browned.

9. With a slotted spoon, transfer the beef and orange strips right into a bowl.

10. With a paper towel, wipe out the skillet.

11. In a similar skillet, heat remaining oil on medium-high heat.

12. Add jalapeño pepper and string beans and stir fry for about 3-4 minutes.

13. Meanwhile add arrowroot powder in reserved marinade and stir to mix.

14. In the skillet, add marinade mixture, beef and bok choy and cook for about 1-2 minutes.

15. Serve hot with garnishing of sesame seeds.

Beef with Asparagus & Bell Pepper

Yield: 4-5 servings
Preparation Time: fifteen minutes
Cooking Time: 13 minutes

Ingredients:

- 4 garlic cloves, minced
- 3 tablespoons coconut aminos
- 1/8 teaspoon red pepper flakes, crushed
- 1/8 teaspoon ground ginger
- Freshly ground black pepper, to taste
- 1 bunch asparagus, trimmed and halved
- 2 tablespoons olive oil, divided
- 1 pound flank steak, trimmed and sliced thinly
- 1 red bell pepper, seeded and sliced
- 3 tablespoons water
- 2 teaspoons arrowroot powder

Directions:

1. In a bowl, mix together garlic, coconut aminos, red pepper flakes, crushed, ground ginger and black pepper. Keep aside.
2. In a pan of boiling water, cook asparagus for about 2 minutes.
3. Drain and rinse under cold water.
4. In a substantial skillet, heat 1 tablespoon of oil on medium-high heat.
5. Add beef and stir fry for around 3-4 minutes.
6. With a slotted spoon, transfer the beef in a bowl.
7. In a similar skillet, heat remaining oil on medium heat.
8. Add asparagus and bell pepper and stir fry for approximately 2-3 minutes.

9. Meanwhile in the bowl, mix together water and arrowroot powder.
10. Stir in beef, garlic mixture and arrowroot mixture and cook for around 3-4 minutes or till desired thickness.

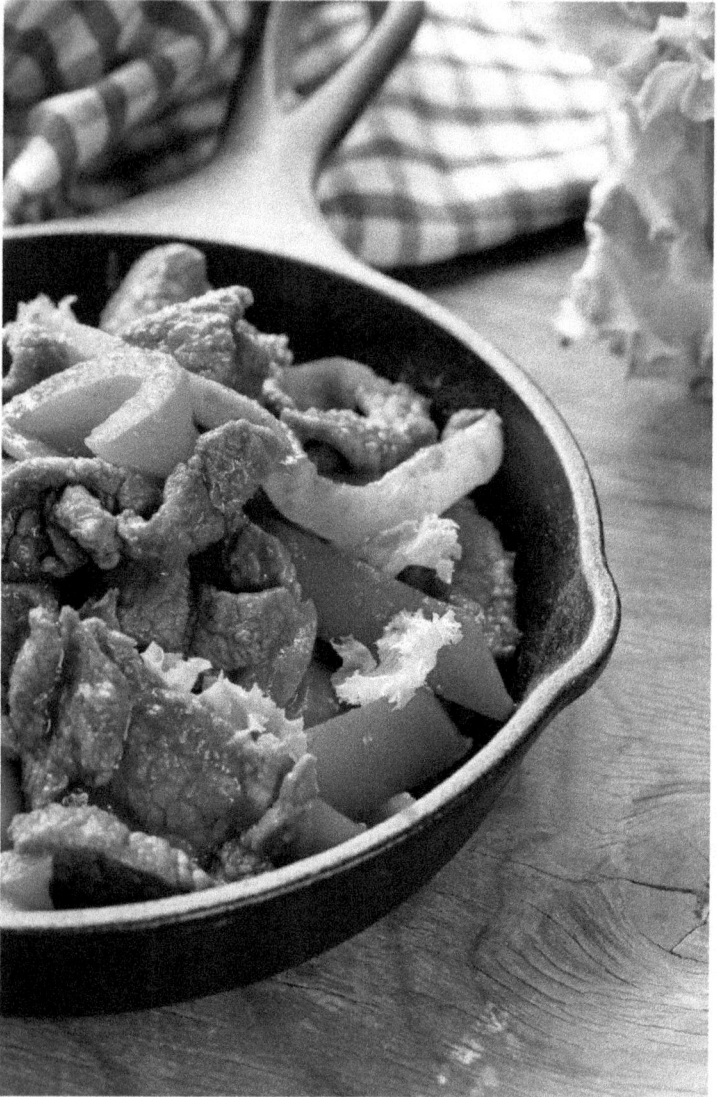

66

Ground Beef with Cabbage

Yield: 6 servings
Preparation Time: 10 minutes
Cooking Time: quarter-hour

Ingredients:
- 1 tbsp olive oil
- 1 onion, sliced thinly
- 2 teaspoons fresh ginger, minced
- 4 garlic cloves, minced
- 1 pound lean ground beef
- 1½ tablespoons fish sauce
- 2 tablespoons fresh lime juice
- 1 small head purple cabbage, shredded
- 2 tablespoons peanut butter
- ½ cup fresh cilantro, chopped

Directions:
1. In a large skillet, heat oil on medium heat.
2. Add onion, ginger and garlic and sauté for about 4-5 minutes.
3. Add beef and cook for approximately 7-8 minutes, getting into pieces using the spoon.
4. Drain off the extra liquid in the skillet.
5. Stir in fish sauce and lime juice and cook for approximately 1 minute.
6. Add cabbage and cook approximately 4-5 minutes or till desired doneness.
7. Stir in peanut butter and cilantro and cook for about 1 minute.
8. Serve hot.

Ground Beef with Cashews & Veggies

Yield: 4 servings
Preparation Time: 15 minutes
Cooking Time: quarter-hour

Ingredients:
- 1½ pound lean ground beef
- 1 tablespoon garlic, minced
- 2 tablespoons fresh ginger, minced
- ¼ cup coconut aminos
- Salt and freshly ground black pepper, to taste
- 1 medium onion, sliced
- 1 can water chestnuts, drained and sliced
- 1 large green bell pepper, seeded and sliced
- ½ cup raw cashews, toasted

Directions:
1. Heat a nonstick skillet on medium-high heat.
2. Add beef and cook for about 6-8 minutes breaking into pieces with the spoon.
3. Add garlic, ginger, coconut aminos, salt and black pepper and cook for approximately 2 minutes.
4. Add vegetables and cook approximately 5 minutes or till desired doneness.
5. Stir in cashews and immediately remove from heat.
6. Serve hot.

Beef & Veggies Chili

Yield: 6-8 servings
Preparation Time: 15 minutes
Cooking Time: one hour

Ingredients:
- 2 pounds lean ground beef
- ½ head cauliflower, chopped into large pieces
- 1 onion, chopped
- 6 garlic cloves, minced
- 2 cups pumpkin puree
- 1 teaspoon dried oregano, crushed
- 1 teaspoon dried thyme, crushed
- 1 teaspoon ground cumin
- 1 teaspoon ground turmeric
- 1-2 teaspoons chili powder
- 1 teaspoon paprika
- 1 teaspoon cayenne pepper
- ¼ teaspoon red pepper flakes, crushed
- Salt and freshly ground black pepper, to taste
- 1 (26-ounce) can tomatoes, drained
- ½ cup water
- 1 cup beef broth

Directions:
1. Heat a substantial pan on medium-high heat.
2. Add beef and stir fry for around 5 minutes.
3. Add cauliflower, onion and garlic and stir fry for approximately 5 minutes.
4. Add spices and herbs and stir to mix well.
5. Stir in remaining ingredients and provide to a boil.

6. Reduce heat to low and simmer, covered approximately 30-45 minutes.

7. Serve hot.

Spicy & Creamy Ground Beef Curry

Yield: 4 servings
Preparation Time: quarter-hour
Cooking Time: 32 minutes

Ingredients:
- 1-2 tablespoons coconut oil
- 1 teaspoon black mustard seeds
- 2 sprigs curry leaves
- 1 Serrano pepper, minced
- 1 large red onion, chopped finely
- 1 (1- inch) piece fresh ginger, minced
- 4 garlic cloves, minced
- 1 teaspoon ground coriander
- 1 teaspoon ground cumin
- ½ teaspoon ground turmeric
- ¼ teaspoon red chili powder
- Salt, to taste
- 1 pound lean ground beef
- 1 potato, peeled and chopped
- 3 medium carrots, peeled and chopped
- ¼ cup water
- 1 (14-ounce) can coconut milk
- Salt and freshly ground black pepper, to taste
- Chopped fresh cilantro, for garnishing

Directions:
1. In a big pan, melt coconut oil on medium heat.

2. Add mustard seeds and sauté for about thirty seconds.

3. Add curry leaves and Serrano pepper and sauté approximately half a minute.

4. Add onion, ginger and garlic and sauté for about 4-5 minutes.
5. Add spices and cook for about 1 minute.
6. Add beef and cook for about 4-5 minutes.
7. Stir in potato, carrot and water and provide with a gentle simmer.
8. Simmer, covered for around 5 minutes.
9. Stir in coconut milk and simmer for around fifteen minutes.
10. Stir in salt and black pepper and remove from heat.
11. Serve hot while using garnishing of cilantro.

Beef Meatballs in Tomato Gravy

Yield: 4 servings
Preparation Time: 20 minutes
Cooking Time: 37 minutes

Ingredients:
For Meatballs:
- 1 pound lean ground beef
- 1 organic egg, bea10
- 1 tablespoon fresh ginger, minced
- 1 garlic oil, minced
- 2 tablespoons fresh cilantro, chopped finely
- 2 tablespoons tomato paste
- 1/3 cup almond meal
- 1 tablespoon ground cumin
- Pinch of ground cinnamon
- Salt and freshly ground black pepper, to taste
- ¼ cup coconut oil

For Tomato Gravy:
- 2 tablespoons coconut oil
- ½ of small onion, chopped
- 2 garlic cloves, chopped
- 1 teaspoon fresh lemon zest, grated finely
- 2 cups tomatoes, chopped finely
- Pinch of ground cinnamon
- 1 teaspoon red pepper flakes, crushed
- ¾ cup chicken broth
- Salt and freshly ground black pepper, to taste
- ¼ cup fresh parsley, chopped

Directions:

1. For meatballs in a sizable bowl, add all ingredients except oil and mix till well combined.
2. Make about 1-inch sized balls from mixture.
3. In a substantial skillet, melt coconut oil on medium heat.
4. Add meatballs and cook for approximately 3-5 minutes or till golden brown all sides.
5. Transfer the meatballs into a bowl.
6. For gravy in a big pan, melt coconut oil on medium heat.
7. Add onion and garlic and sauté approximately 4 minutes.
8. Add lemon zest and sauté approximately 1 minute.
9. Add tomatoes, cinnamon, red pepper flakes and broth and simmer approximately 7 minutes.
10. Stir in salt, black pepper and meatballs and reduce the warmth to medium-low.
11. Simmer for approximately twenty minutes.
12. Serve hot with all the garnishing of parsley.

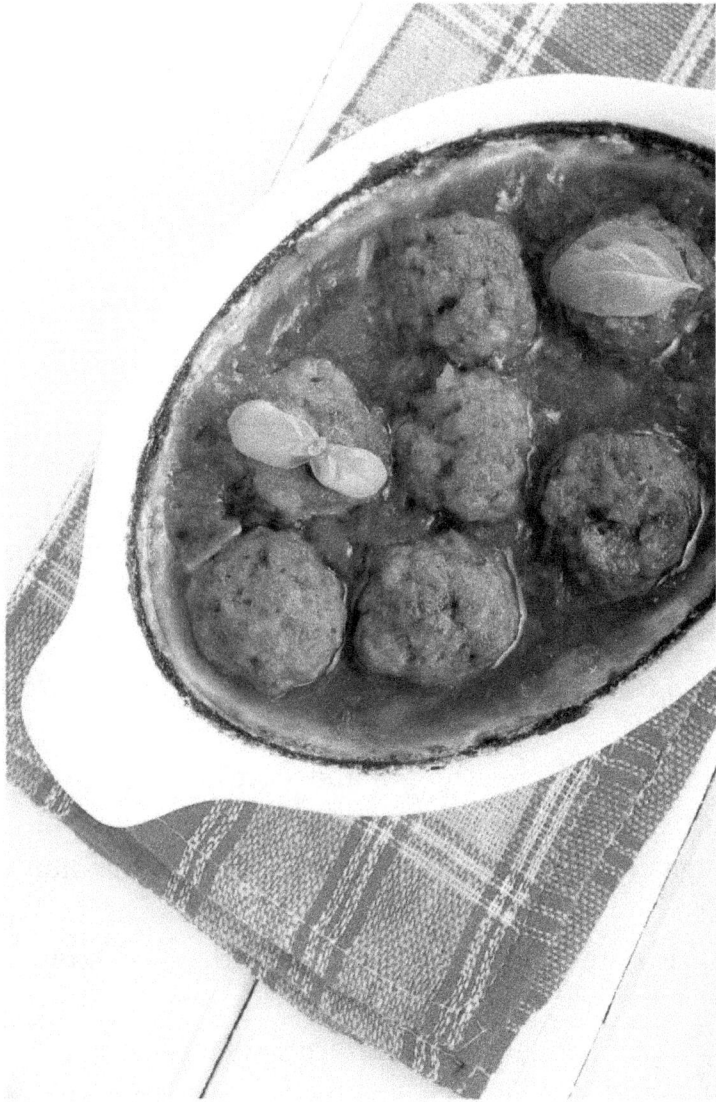

Pan Grilled Flank Steak

Yield: 3-4 servings
Preparation Time: 10 minutes
Cooking Time: 12-16 minutes

Ingredients:
- 8 medium garlic cloves, crushed
- 1 (5-inch) piece fresh ginger, sliced thinly
- 1 tablespoon organic honey
- ¼ cup organic olive oil
- Salt and freshly ground black pepper, to taste
- 1½ pound flank steak, trimmed

Directions:
1. In a large sealable bag, mix together all ingredients except steak.
2. Add steak and coat with marinade generously.
3. Seal the bag and refrigerate to marinate for approximately one day.
4. Remove from refrigerator and leave at room temperature for approximately 15 minutes.
5. Lightly, grease a grill pan as well as heat to medium-high heat.
6. Discard the surplus marinade from the steak and place in grill pan.
7. Cook for about 6-8 minutes from each party.
8. Remove from grill pan and keep aside for around 10 min before slicing.
9. With a clear, crisp knife cut into desired slices and serve.

Citrus Poached Salmon

Yield: 3 servings
Preparation Time: fifteen minutes
Cooking Time: 12 minutes

Ingredients:

- 3 garlic cloves, crushed
- 1½ teaspoons fresh ginger, grated finely
- 1/3 cup fresh orange juice
- 3 tablespoons coconut aminos
- 3 (6-ounce) salmon fillets

Directions:

1. In a bowl, mix together all ingredients except salmon.

2. In the bottom of your large pan, squeeze salmon fillet.

3. Place the ginger mixture in the salmon and aside for about quarter-hour.

4. Place the pan on high heat and convey to your boil.

5. Reduce the heat to low and simmer, covered for about 10-12 minutes or till desired doneness.

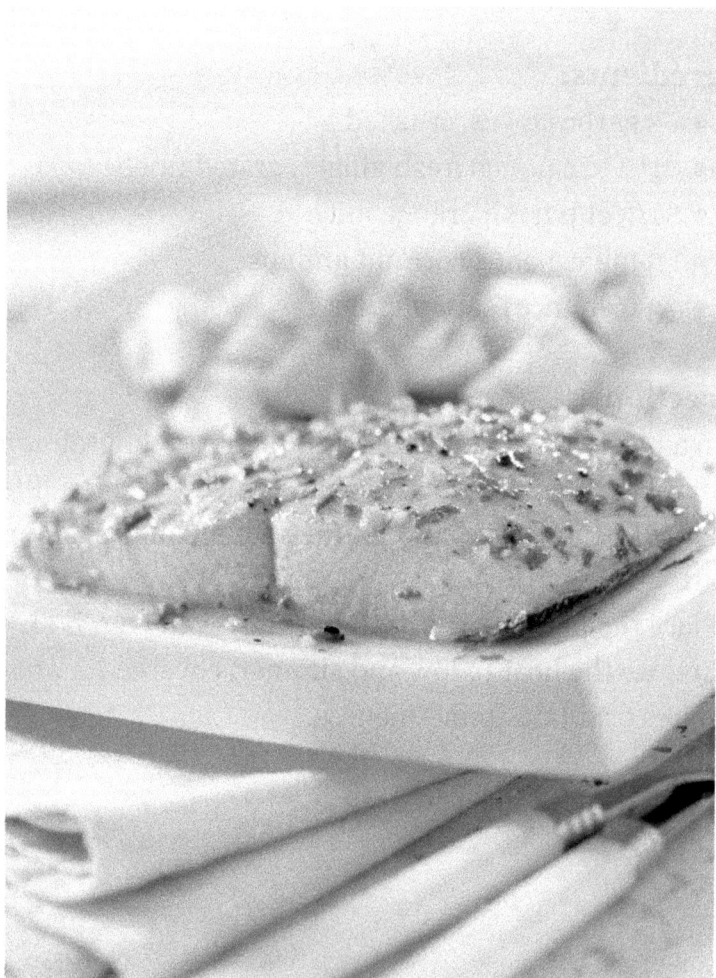

Broiled Spicy Salmon

Yield: 4 servings
Preparation Time: fifteen minutes
Cooking Time: 14 minutes

Ingredients:
- ¼ cup low- Fat plain Greek yogurt
- ½ teaspoon ground coriander
- ½ teaspoon ground turmeric
- ½ teaspoon ground ginger
- ¼ tsp cayenne pepper
- Salt and freshly ground black pepper, to taste
- 4 (6-ounce) skinless salmon fillets

Directions:
1. Heat the broiler of the oven. Grease a broiler pan.
2. In a bowl, mix together all ingredients except the salmon.
3. Arrange salmon fillets onto prepared broiler pan inside a single layer.
4. Place the yogurt mixture over each fillet evenly.
5. Broil approximately 12-14 minutes.
6. Serve immediately.

Baked Sweet Lemony Salmon

Yield: 2 servings
Preparation Time: 15 minutes
Cooking Time: 12 minutes

Ingredients:

- 2 (8-ounce) salmon fillets
- ½ teaspoon organic honey and even more for drizzling
- 1/3 teaspoon ground turmeric, divided
- Freshly ground black pepper, to taste
- 2 large lemon slices

Directions:

1. In a zip lock bag, add salmon, ½ teaspoon of honey, ¼ teaspoon of turmeric and black pepper.
2. Seal the bag and shake to coat well.
3. Refrigerate to marinate for around 1 hour.
4. Preheat the oven to 40 degrees F.
5. Transfer the salmon fillets onto a cookie sheet in the single layer.
6. Cover the fillets with marinade.
7. Place the salmon fillets, skin-side up and bake for around 6 minutes.
8. Carefully, customize the side of fillets.
9. Sprinkle with remaining turmeric and black pepper evenly.
10. Place 1 lemon slice over each fillet and drizzle with honey.
11. Bake for approximately 6 minutes.

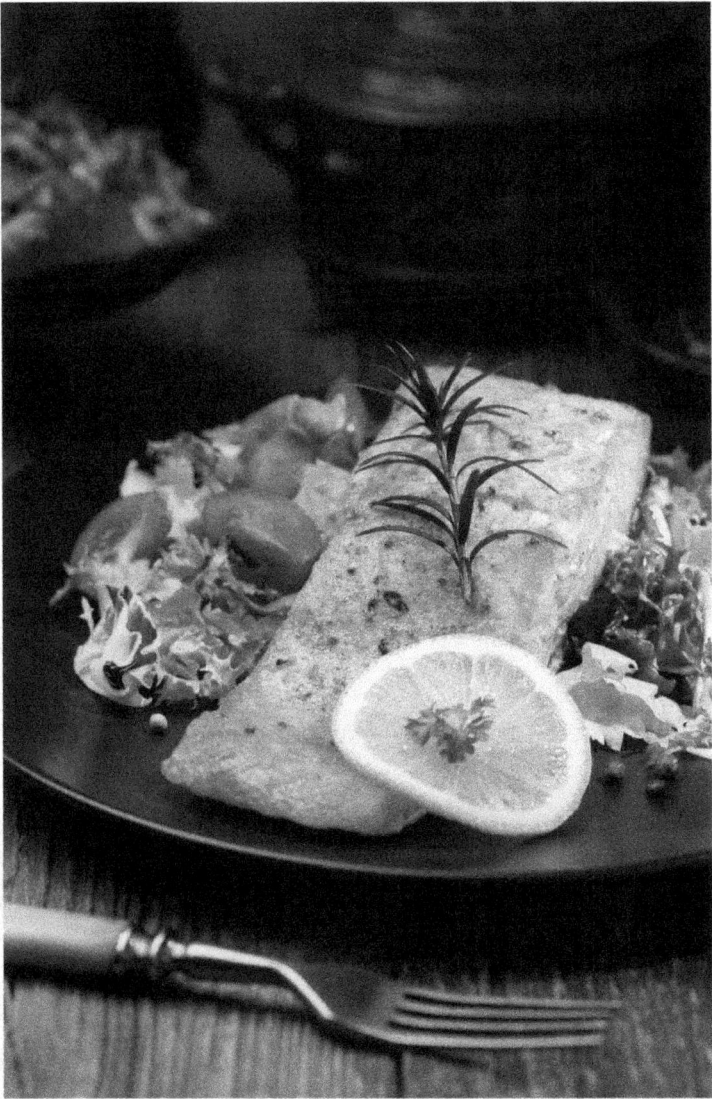

Chicken with Veggie Combo

Yield: 2 servings
Preparation Time: 25 minutes
Cooking Time: fifteen minutes

Ingredients:
- 1 tbsp olive oil
- 1 large skinless, boneless chicken white meat, cubed
- 1 cup small cauliflower florets
- 1 cup fresh shiitake mushrooms, sliced
- 1 cup bok choy, chopped
- 1 cup carrot, peeled and spiralized Blade C
- ½ teaspoon ground ginger
- ½ teaspoon garlic salt
- 1 large zucchini, spiralized Blade C

Directions:
1. In a big skillet, heat oil on medium-high heat.
2. Add chicken and stir fry approximately 2 minutes or till golden brown.
3. Add onion and cabbage and cook for around 4-5 minutes.
4. Add cauliflower whilst without stirring for around 30-45 seconds.
5. Cook, tossing occasionally for about2 minutes.
6. Add mushrooms and cook for approximately 2 minutes.
7. Add bok choy, carrot, ground ginger and garlic salt and cook, tossing occasionally or about 2-3 minutes.
8. Add zucchini and cook for around 2-3 minutes.
9. Remove from heat and make aside for about 3-5 minutes before serving.

Chicken with Mango, Veggies & Cashews

Yield: 4 servings
Preparation Time: 25 minutes
Cooking Time: 18 minutes

Ingredients:
- 2 tablespoons coconut oil
- 2 skinless, boneless chicken breasts, sliced
- 1 red onion, sliced thinly
- 2 minced garlic cloves
- 2 tablespoons fresh ginger, minced
- 1 ripe mango, peeled, pitted and cubed
- 1 bunch broccoli, cut into small florets
- 1 zucchini, sliced
- 1 cup mushrooms, sliced
- 1 red bell pepper, seeded and cubed
- 2 cups beans sprouts
- 3 tablespoons coconut aminos
- ¼ teaspoon red chili flakes, crushed
- Salt and freshly ground black pepper, to taste
- ¼ cup cashews, toasted

Directions:
1. In a big skillet, melt coconut oil on medium-high heat.
2. Add chicken and stir fry for approximately 4-5 minutes or till golden brown.
3. Transfer chicken to a plate.
4. In the same skillet, add onion, garlic and ginger and sauté for about 1-2 minutes.

5. Add mango, broccoli, zucchini and bell pepper and cook for approximately 5-7 minutes.

6. Add chicken, beans sprouts, coconut aminos, red chili flakes, salt and black pepper and cook for approximately 3-4 minutes or till desired doneness.

7. Serve with the topping of cashews.

Chicken in Spicy Gravy

Yield: 3-4 servings
Preparation Time: 10 min
Cooking Time: 38 minutes

Ingredients:
For Marinade:
- 1 teaspoon garlic paste
- 1 teaspoon ginger paste
- 2 teaspoons chili powder
- ½ teaspoon ground turmeric
- Salt, to taste
- 1 teaspoon freshly squeezed lemon juice
- Water, as required
- 1 pound skinless, boneless chicken breast, cut into medium pieces

For Cooking:
- 5 tbsp essential olive oil
- 2 large onions, sliced thinly
- 10 curry leaves
- 1½ teaspoons garlic paste
- 1½ teaspoons ginger paste
- 2 green chilies, chopped
- 2 teaspoons ground coriander
- 1 teaspoon garam masala
- 1 teaspoon chili powder
- 1 teaspoon ground turmeric
- Salt and freshly ground black pepper, to taste
- ½ cup chicken broth

- 1 large tomato, chopped finely

Directions:
1. For marinade, in a big bowl mix together all ingredients except water and chicken.
2. Add enough water and mix till a paste forms.
3. Add chicken and coat with marinade generously.
4. Cover and refrigerate to marinate for around 30 minutes.
5. In a big skillet, heat oil on medium-high heat.
6. Add chicken and stir fry approximately 4-5 minutes or till golden brown.
7. Transfer chicken to a plate.
8. In a similar skillet, add onion and curry leaves on medium-low heat.
9. Cook, covered for around 15-20 minutes till golden brown, stirring occasionally.
10. Add garlic ginger paste and green chilies and sauté approximately 1-2 minutes.
11. Stir in spices and sauté for approximately 1 minute.
12. Stir in chicken and cook covered for approximately 5-6 minutes.
13. Add broth and cook for approximately 5-6 minutes.
14. Add tomato and cook, stirring occasionally approximately 5 minutes more.

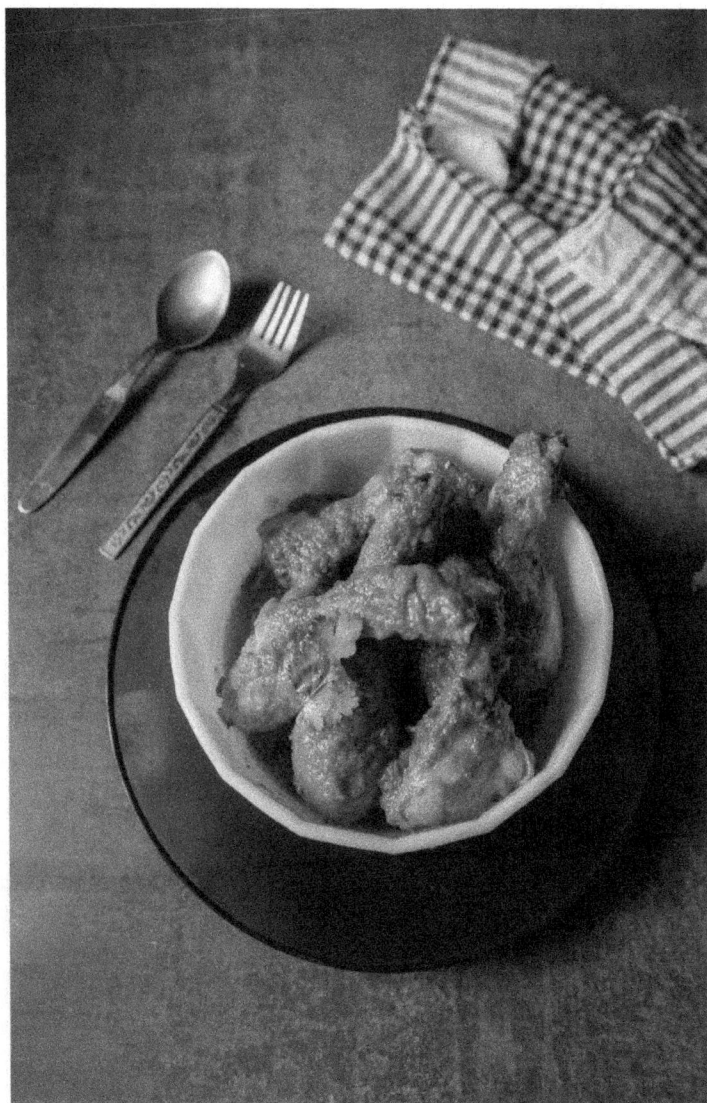

Citrus Glazed Chicken

Yield: 6 servings
Preparation Time: 10 min
Cooking Time: 18 minutes

Ingredients:
- 3 garlic cloves, minced
- ½ cup fresh orange juice
- 1 tablespoon apple cider vinegar
- 2 tablespoons coconut aminos
- ½ teaspoon orange blossom water
- ¼ teaspoon ground ginger
- ¼ teaspoon ground cinnamon
- Salt, to taste
- 2 pound skinless, bone-in chicken thighs

Directions:

1. For marinade, in a big bowl mix together all ingredients except chicken.
2. Add chicken and coat with marinade generously.
3. Cover and refrigerate to marinate for around 2 hours.
4. Heat a sizable nonstick skillet, on medium-high heat.
5. Add chicken in skillet, reserving marinade.
6. Cook for about 5-6 minutes or till golden brown.
7. Flip the medial side and cook for about 4 minutes.
8. Add reserved marinade and provide to a boil.
9. Reduce heat to medium-low heat.
10. Cook, covered for about 6-8 minutes or till sauce becomes thick.
11. Serve warm.

Chicken with Chickpeas & Veggies

Yield: 4 servings
Preparation Time: 15 minutes
Cooking Time: 36 minutes

Ingredients:

- 1 pound skinless, boneless chicken, cubed
- Salt, to taste
- 2 carrots, peeled and sliced
- 1 onion, chopped
- 2 celery stalks, chopped
- 2 garlic cloves, chopped
- 1 tablespoon fresh ginger root, minced
- ½ teaspoon dried oregano, crushed
- ¾ teaspoon ground cumin
- ½ teaspoon paprika
- ¼ tsp red pepper cayenne
- ¼ teaspoon ground turmeric
- 1 cup tomatoes, crushed
- 1½ cups chicken broth
- 1 zucchini, sliced
- 1 cup canned chickpeas, drained
- 1 tablespoon freshly squeezed lemon juice

Directions:

1. Heat a big nonstick pan on medium heat.
2. Add chicken and sprinkle with salt and cook for approximately 4-5 minutes.
3. With a slotted spoon, transfer chicken right into a plate.
4. In exactly the same pan, add carrot, onion, celery and garlic and sauté for about 4-5 minutes.

5. Add ginger, oregano and spices and sauté for around 1 minute.

6. Add chicken, tomato and broth and provide to some boil.

7. Reduce the temperature to low and simmer for approximately 10 minutes.

8. Add zucchini and chickpeas and simmer, covered for approximately fifteen minutes.

9. Stir in fresh lemon juice and serve hot.

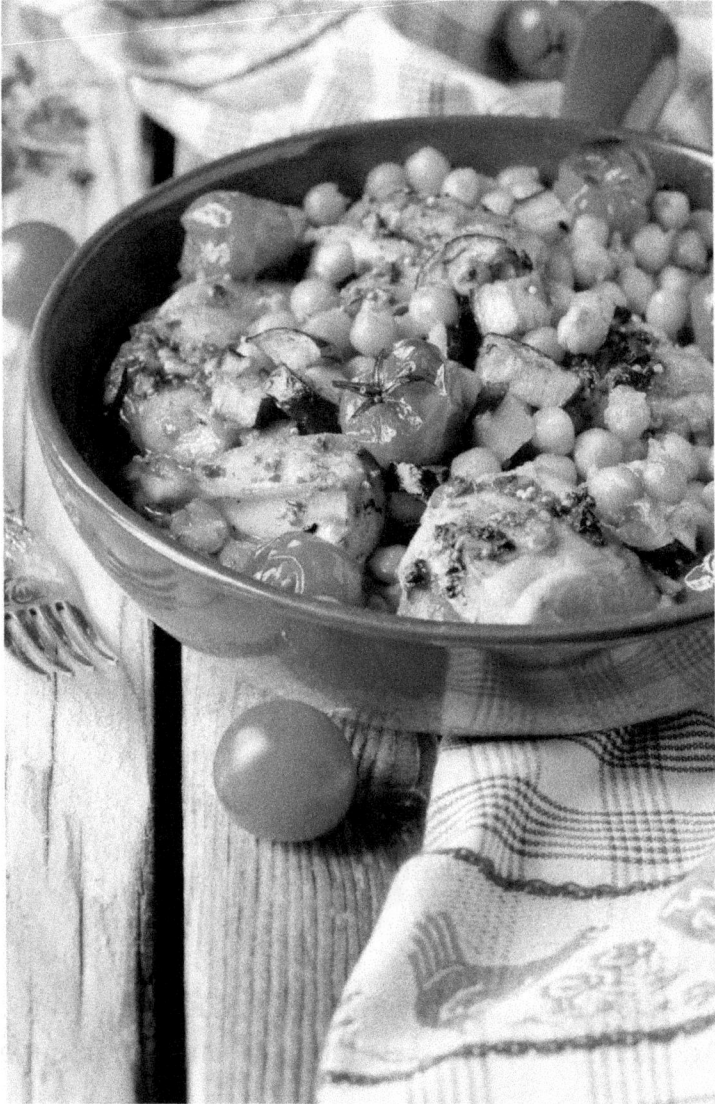

Chicken Chili with Sweet Potato

Yield: 6 servings
Preparation Time: 15 minutes
Cooking Time: 35 minutes

Ingredients:

- 2 tablespoons extra-virgin essential olive oil
- 1 medium red onion, chopped
- 4- 6 garlic cloves, minced
- 2 medium sweet potatoes, peeled and cubed
- 2 teaspoons dried oregano, crushed
- 2 teaspoons ground cumin
- 2 teaspoons ground ginger
- 1 teaspoon red chili powder
- ¼ teaspoon red pepper flakes, crushed
- Salt, to taste
- 4 cups chicken broth
- 2 (15-ounce) cans white beans, rinsed and drained
- ¾ cup mild roasted green chiles
- 4 cups cooked chicken, shredded
- 1 tablespoon fresh lime juice
- 2 tablespoons fresh cilantro, chopped

Directions:

1. In a substantial pan, heat oil on medium-high heat.
2. Add poblano pepper and onion and sauté for about 2-3 minutes.
3. Add garlic and sauté for approximately 1-2 minutes.
4. Add sweet potato, oregano and spices and stir to combine well.
5. Add broth, beans and green chiles and provide to your boil.

6. Reduce the warmth to low and simmer for about 25-a half-hour.

7. Stir in chicken and lime juice and take off from heat.

8. Serve hot with all the topping of cilantro.

Chicken & Tomato Curry

Yield: 4 servings
Preparation Time: 15 minutes
Cooking Time: 70 minutes

Ingredients:

- 3 tablespoons organic olive oil
- 1 medium onion, chopped
- 1 teaspoon ginger paste
- 1 teaspoon garlic paste
- 4-6 large fresh tomatoes, chopped finely
- 1 teaspoon ground cumin
- Pinch of ground turmeric
- 1½ teaspoons red chili powder
- 2 pounds bone-in chicken breasts, cut each breast into 2-3 pieces
- 2 cups water, divided
- 2 cardamom pods
- 2 tablespoons fresh cilantro, chopped

Directions:

1. In a big pan, heat oil on medium heat.
2. Add onion and sauté for about 8-9 minutes.
3. Add ginger and garlic and sauté for about1 minute.
4. Add tomatoes and spices reducing the heat to medium-low.
5. Cook, stirring occasionally for about 15-20 min.
6. Remove from heat whilst aside to chill slightly.
7. In a blender, add tomato mixture and pulse till smooth.
8. Return the mixture to the pan with chicken and ½ cup from the water on medium-high heat.
Cook, stirring occasionally approximately 15-twenty minutes.

9. Add cardamom pods and remaining water and lower the temperature to low.

10. Simmer for approximately 15-20 min.

11. Serve top with the topping of cilantro.

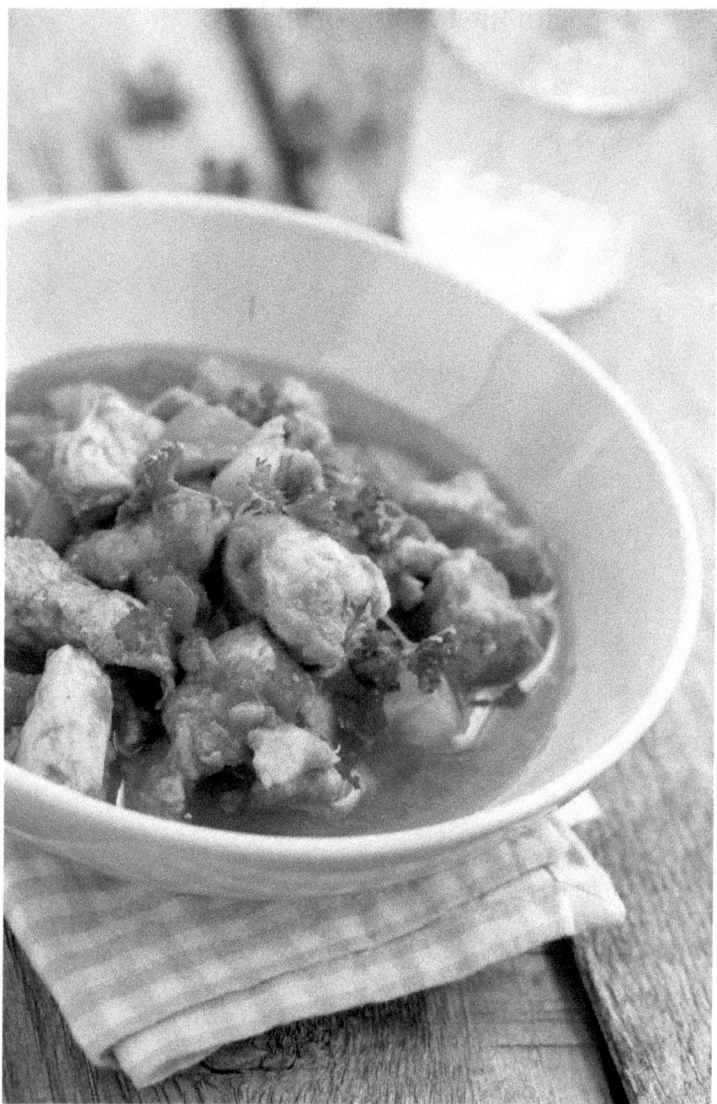

Lemony Fruit Salad

Yield: 16 servings
Preparation Time: 25 minutes

Ingredients:
- 1 fresh pineapple, peeled, cored and chopped
- 2 large mangoes, peeled, pitted and chopped
- 2 large Fuji apples, cored and chopped
- 2 large red Bartlett pears, cored and chopped
- 2 large navel oranges, peeled, seeded and sectioned
- 2 teaspoons fresh ginger, grated finely
- 2 tablespoons organic honey
- ¼ cup fresh lemon juice

Directions:
1. In a big bowl, mix together all fruits.
2. In a little bowl, add remaining ingredients and beat well.
3. Place honey mixture over fruit mixture and toss to coat well.
4. Refrigerate, covered till chilled completely.

Wheat Berries & Mango Salad

Yield: 4 servings
Preparation Time: 20 minutes
Cooking Time: 35 minutes

Ingredients:
For Salad:

- 2 cups water
- 1 cup wheat berries
- 1 mango, peeled, pitted and cubed
- ½ of red bell pepper, seeded and chopped
- 2 scallions, chopped
- ½ cup fresh mint leaves, chopped
- ½ cup cranberries
- ½ cup walnuts, toasted and chopped

For Dressing:

- 1 tablespoon fresh ginger, minced
- 1 cup plain Greek yogurt
- 3 tablespoons raw honey
- ½ teaspoon balsamic vinegar
- Salt and freshly ground black pepper, to taste

Directions:
1. In a pan, add water and warmth berries and bring to your boil.
2. Cover and cook for approximately 35 minutes.
3. Remove from heat whilst aside for cooling.
4. In a large bowl, add wheat berries and remaining ingredients and mix.
5. In a little bowl, add dressing ingredients and beat well.
6. Place dressing over fruit mixture and toss to coat well.
7. Serve immediately.

Berries & Watermelon Salad

Yield: 8-10 servings
Preparation Time: 20 min

Ingredients:

- 2½ pound seedless watermelon, cubed
- 2 cartons fresh strawberries, hulled and sliced
- 2 cups fresh blueberries
- 1 tablespoon fresh ginger root, grated
- ¼- ounce fresh mint leaves, chopped
- 1 tablespoon raw honey
- ¼ cup fresh lime juice

Directions:

1. In a sizable bowl, mix together all ingredients.
2. Serve immediately.

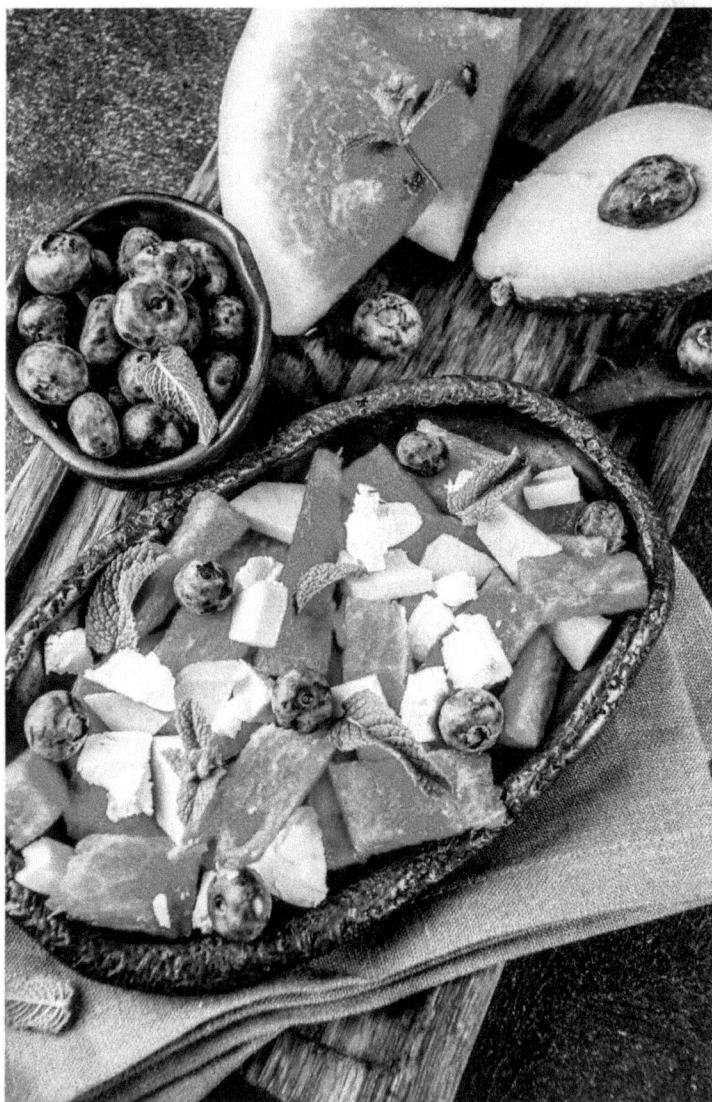

Pear & Jicama Salad

Yield: 4 servings
Preparation Time: quarter-hour

Ingredients:
For Salad:
- 2 small pears, cored and sliced thinly
- 1 pound jicama, sliced into matchsticks
- 1 sprig fresh mint
- 1 sprig fresh parsley

For Dressing:
- 2 tablespoons extra virgin olive oil
- 3 tablespoons fresh orange juice
- 1 tablespoon using apple cider vinegar
- ¼ teaspoon ginger powder
- Salt, to taste

Directions:
1. In a big bowl, mix together all salad ingredients.
2. In a smaller bowl, add dressing ingredients and beat well.
3. Place dressing over salad mixture and toss to coat well.
4. Serve immediately.

Carrot & Almond Salad

Yield: 4 servings
Preparation Time: 15 minutes

Ingredients:
- 1 garlic clove, minced
- 2 teaspoons fresh ginger, grated finely
- ¼ cup coconut milk
- 2 tablespoons almond butter
- 2 tablespoons coconut aminos
- 1 tablespoon fresh lemon juice
- Pinch of cayenne
- Salt, to taste
- 5 large carrots, peeled and grated
- Chopped almonds, to taste

Directions:
1. In a large bowl, add all ingredients except carrots and almonds and mix till well combined.
2. Add carrots and stir to mix.
3. Serve with the garnishing of almonds.

Beet, Carrot & Parsley Salad

Yield: 5 servings
Preparation Time: 15 minutes

Ingredients:
For Salad:
- 1 cup Daikon radishes, trimmed, peeled and julienned
- 3 cups carrots, peeled and julienned
- ½ cup fresh parsley, chopped

For Dressing:
- 1 teaspoon fresh ginger, grated finely
- 2 tablespoons balsamic vinegar
- 1 tablespoon extra-virgin extra virgin olive oil
- 2 teaspoons coconut aminos
- 2 teaspoons raw honey
- ¼ teaspoon granulated garlic
- Salt, to taste

Directions:
1. In a big bowl, mix together all salad ingredients.
2. In a tiny bowl, add dressing ingredients and beat well.
3. Place dressing over fruit mixture and toss to coat well.
4. Serve immediately.

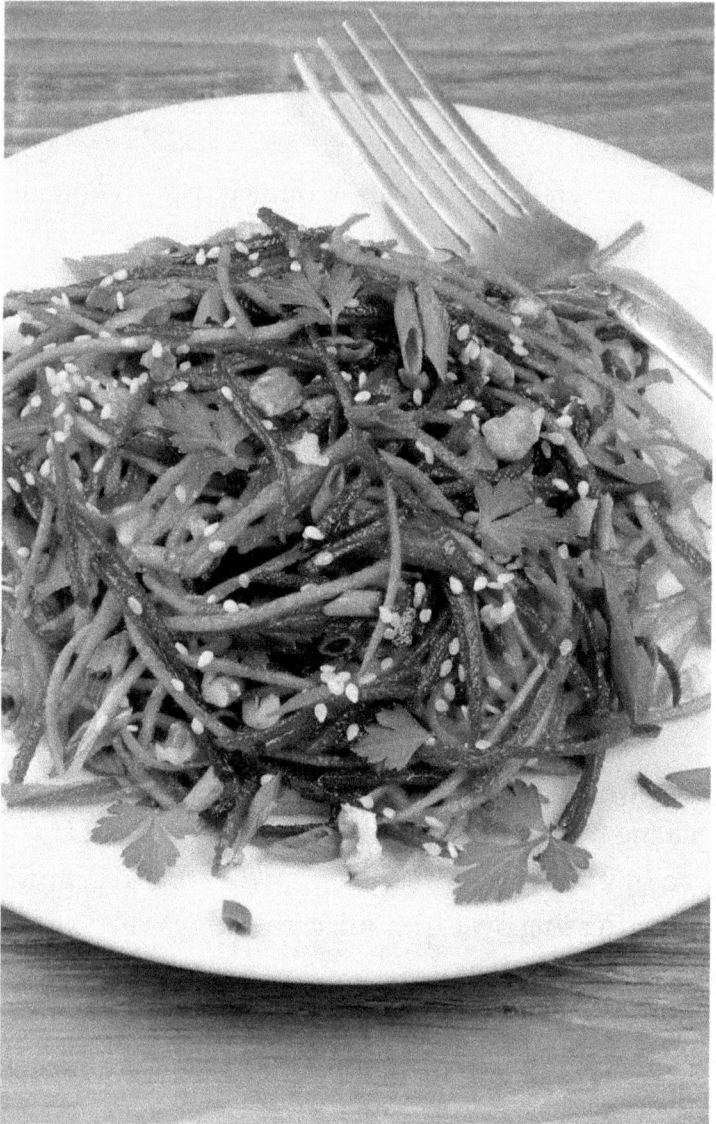

Greens & Seeds Salad

Yield: 4 servings
Preparation Time: 20 minutes
Cooking Time: 6 minutes

Ingredients:

- 1½ teaspoons fresh ginger, grated finely
- 2 tablespoons apple cider vinegar treatment
- 3 tablespoons olive oil
- 1 teaspoon sesame oil, toasted
- 3 teaspoons raw honey, divided
- ½ teaspoon red pepper flakes, crushed and divided
- Salt, to taste
- 1 tablespoon water
- 2 tablespoons raw sunflower seeds
- 1 tablespoon raw sesame seeds
- 1 tablespoon raw pumpkin seeds
- 10-ounce collard greens, stems and ribs removed and thinly sliced leaves

Directions:

1. For dressing, inside a bowl add ginger, vinegar, both oils, 1 teaspoon of honey, ¼ teaspoon red pepper flakes and salt and bat till well combined. Keep aside.
2. In another bowl, add remaining honey, remaining red pepper flakes and water and mix till well combined.
3. Heat a medium nonstick skillet on medium heat.
4. Add all seeds and cook, stirring for approximately 3 minutes.
5. Stir in honey mixture and cook, stirring continuously for about 3 minutes.

6. Transfer the seeds mixture onto a parchment paper and set aside to cool down completely.

7. Break the seeds mixture into small pieces.

8. In a large bowl, add the greens, 2 teaspoons with the dressing plus a little salt and toss to coat well.

9. With both your hands, rub the greens for around a few seconds.

10. Add remaining dressing and toss to coat well.

11. Serve with a garnish of seeds pieces.

Notes

www.ingramcontent.com/pod-product-compliance
Lightning Source LLC
Chambersburg PA
CBHW050800030426
42336CB00012B/1881